Resource Compendium Available for Cervical and Breast Cancer Control and Prevention in the Majority World: Focus on the Caribbean, Mexico, Central and South America

Resource Compendium Available for Cervical and Breast Cancer Control and Prevention in the Majority World: Focus on the Caribbean, Mexico, Central and South America

Laurie Elit
Juravinski Cancer Centre, Hamilton, Ontario, Canada
Editor

Nova Biomedical Books
New York

For permission to use material from this book please contact us:
Telephone 631-231-7269; Fax 631-231-8175
Web Site: http://www.novapublishers.com

LIBRARY OF CONGRESS CATALOGING-IN-PUBLICATION DATA

Elit, Laurie.
Compendium of resources available for cervix and breast cancer care in the majority world / Laurie Elit (author). p. ; cm.
Includes index.
ISBN-13: 978-1-60021-844-6 (hardcover)
ISBN-10: 1-60021-844-X (hardcover)
1. Cervix uteri--Cancer--Information services--Directories. 2. Breast--Cancer--Information services--Directories. 3. Cervix uteri--Cancer--Research--Directories 4. Breast--Cancer--Research--Directories. 5. Cervix uteri--Cancer--Bibliography. 6. Breast--Cancer--Bibliography. I. Title. [DNLM: 1. Uterine Cervical Neoplasms--Bibliography. 2. Uterine Cervical Neoplasms--Directory. 3. Uterine Cervical Neoplasms--Resource Guides. 4. Breast Neoplasms--Bibliography. 5. Breast Neoplasms--Directory. 6. Breast Neoplasms--Resource Guides. WP 22.1 E47c 2007] RC280.U8E44 2007
616.99'466--dc22 2007025692

Published by Nova Science Publishers, Inc. ✣ New York

CONTENTS

PREFACE

Cervix Cancer is the second leading cause of death for women world-wide. The rates of breast cancer are quickly rising through out the world. In part these dismal statistics are related to the fact that disease in low resource countries is identified in advanced stages when cure is improbable. Cervix and breast cancer are preventable or at least curable when identified earlier. This can happen when screening programs are in place. This compendium provide references to the international agencies and societies involved in dealing with this problem, research conducted on breast and cervical cancer prevention and control in the low resource countries of the Western hemisphere and educational resources available for cancer control planner through to the public.

ACKNOWLEDGEMENT

This resource is one product of my 2006 sabbatical at the National Cancer Institute, Bethesda Maryland. This opportunity was funded in part by a MacKenzie Fellowship in Surgery and a Clinical Traineeship Grant from the Royal College of Physicians and Surgeons Canada.

Chapter 1

CERVICAL CANCER

SECTION 1: AGENCIES AND SOCIETIES INVOLVED IN CERVIX CANCER WORK IN THE MAJORITY WORLD

We have indicated where information was available whether the society or agency had regional representation from the majority world on their board or whether they had branch offices in countries of the majority world

Agency	**Majority world representation on their board or branch offices in majority world countres**	**Weblink**	**Contact**
United Nations			
IAEA International Atomic Energy Agency	Yes	http://www.iaea.org/	International Atomic Energy Agency P.O. Box 100 Wagramer Strasse 5 A-1400 Vienna, Austria Tel: (+431) 2600-0 Fax: (+431) 2600-7 IAEA Office at the United Nations 1 United Nations Plaza Room DC-1-1155 New York, NY 10017 USA Tel: (001) 212-963-6010 or 6011 Fax: (001) 917-367-4046 IAEA Office in Geneva United Nations Room B 426 Palais des Nations CH-1211 Geneva 10

			Switzerland Tel: (+41-22) 917-3632 Fax: (+41-22) 917-0066
PACT Programme of Action for Cancer Treatment		http://www-naweb.iaea.org/pact/	Mr. Massoud Samiei PACT Programme Manager International Atomic Energy Agency P.O. Box 100 Wagramer Strasse 5 A-1400 Vienna, Austria pact@iaea.org
World Health Organization			
WHO : World Health Organization	Yes	http://who.int	Avenue Appia 20 1211 Geneva 27 Switzerland Telephone: (+ 41 22) 791 21 11 Facsimile (fax): (+ 41 22) 791 3111 Telex: 415 416 Telegraph: UNISANTE GENEVA
IARC: International Agency for Research in Cancer		http://www.iarc.fr/	IARC 150 Cours Albert-Thomas 69372 Lyon Cedex 08 France Tel +33 (0) 472738485 FAX 33 (0) 472738575
Regional Office for PAHO: PanAmerican Health Organization		http://www.paho.org/	Regional Office for the Americas 525, 23rd Street, N.W. Washington, DC 20037 USA Telephone: +1 202 974 3000 Facsimile: +1 202 974 3663 E-mail: postmaster@paho.org Regional Director: Dr Mirta Roses
Regional Office for Africa		http://www.afro.who.int/	Regional Office for Africa Cite du Djoue, P.O.Box 06 Brazzaville Congo Telephone: + 242 839 100 / +47 241 39100 Facsimile: + 242 839 501 / +47 241 395018 E-mail: regafro@whoafr.org Regional Director: Dr L. Sambo

Regional Office for South-East Asia		http://www.searo.who.int/	Regional Office for South-East Asia World Health House Indraprastha Estate Mahatama Gandhi Marg New Delhi 110 002 India Telephone: + 91-11-2337 0804 Facsimile: + 91-11-2337 9507 E-mail: pandeyh@whosea.org Regional Director: Dr Samlee Plianbangchang
Regional Office for Europe		http://www.euro.who.int/	Regional Office for Europe 8, Scherfigsvej DK-2100 Copenhagen 0, Denmark Telephone: + 45 39 171 717 Facsimile: + 45 39 171 818 E-mail: postmaster@euro.who.int Regional Director: Marc Danzon
Regional Office for Eastern Mediterranean		http://www.emro.who.int/	Regional Office for the Eastern Mediterranean Abdul Razzak Al Sanhouri Street, P.O. Box 7608, Nasr City, Cairo 11371, Egypt Telephone: + 202 670 25 35 Facsimile: + 202 670 24 92 or 670 24 94 E-mail: postmaster@emro.who.int Regional Director: Dr Hussein Abdel-Razzak Al Gezairy
Regional Office for Western Pacific		http://www.wpro.who.int/	Regional Office for the Western Pacific P.O. Box 2932 1000 Manila Philippines Telephone: + 63 2 528 8001 E-mail: postmaster@wpro.who.int Regional Director: Dr Shigeru Omi

Global Alliances			
ACCP: Alliance for Cervical Cancer Prevention		http://www.alliance-cxca.org/	PATH Alliance coordinating agency 1455 NW Leary Way Seattle, Washington 98107 USA Tel: (206) 285-3500
Governmental Organizations			
CDC: Centres for disease control		http://www.cdc.gov/	Centers for Disease Control and Prevention, 1600 Clifton Rd, Atlanta, GA 30333, U.S.A Tel: (404) 639-3311 / Public Inquiries: (404) 639-3534 / (800) 311-3435
NCI: National Cancer Institute		http://www.cancer.gov/	NCI Public Inquiries Office 6116 Executive Boulevard Room 3036A Bethesda, MD 20892-8322 Tel: 1-800-4-CANCER / (1-800-422-6237)
Nongovernmental organizations			
American Cancer Society (ACS)	No	http://www.cancer.org/docroot/home/index.asp	Tel: 1-800-ACS-2345 (1-866-228-4327)
Cochrane collaboration	No	http://www.cochrane.org/	The Cochrane Collaboration Secretariat Summertown Pavilion 18-24 Middle Way Oxford UK OX2 7LG Phone: +44 1865 310138 Fax: +44 1865 316023
EngenderHealth	20 offices in the field, and more than 70% of our staff work in countries across Asia, Africa, and the Americas.	http://www.engenderhealth.org/	EngenderHealth 440 Ninth Avenue New York, New York 10001 USA Contact: Jan Bradley, M.A. Tel: (212) 561-8000
EUROGIN: European research organization on genital infection and neoplasia	Committee Representation from: Latin America Brazil USA Africa	http://www.eurogin.com/	EUROGIN 174, rue de Courcelles 75017 Paris Tel : +33 1 44 40 01 20 Fax: +33 1 47 66 74 70

	Asia Australia		
Gynecologic Cancer Foundation	No	http://www.thegcf.org/	230 W. Monroe, Suite 2528 Chicago, IL 60606 Tel: (312)578.1439 E-mail: info@thegcf.org Hotline: 800.444.4441
Institute of Medicine	Board on African Science Academy Development (joint with the National Research Council [NRC]); Board on Children, Youth, and Families (joint with NRC); Food and Nutrition Board; Board on Global Health; Board on Health Care Services; Board on Population Health and Public Health Practice; Board on Health Sciences Policy; and Board on Military and Veterans Health.	http://www.iom.edu/	Institute of Medicine 500 Fifth Street NW Washington DC 20001 iomwww@nas.edu Tel: (202)334.2352 Fax: (202)334.1412
International Union Against cancer (UICC)	Yes	http://www.uicc.org	International Union Against Cancer (UICC) 62 route de Frontenex 1207 Geneva; Switzerland Tel +41 22 809 1811 Fax + 41 22 809 1810
International Association for Hospice and Palliative Cancer	No	http://www.hospicecare.com/	*International Association Hospice and Palliative Care* 5535 Memorial Dr. Suite F - PMB 509 Houston TX 77007 USA Tel: +1 (936) 321-9846 Toll Free +1 (866) 374 2472 Fax +1 (713) 880-2948
International Observatory on End of Life	No	http://www.eolc-observatory.net/	Tel: +44 (0)1524 594976.
JHPIEGO, an affiliate of Johns Hopkins University	Field offices in Africa, Asia and Latin America	http://www.jhpiego.org/	JHPIEGO 1615 Thames Street Baltimore, Maryland 21231 USA Tel: (410) 537-1913

PATH: Programme in advanced technologies in Health	Offices in 16 countries	http://www.path.org/	PATH Alliance coordinating agency 1455 NW Leary Way Seattle, Washington 98107 USA Tel: (206) 285-3500
International Societies			
International Academy of Cytology	Yes	http://www.cytology-iac.org/	
International Federation for Cervical Pathology and Colposcopy	Yes	http://www.ifcpc.org/ifcpc/home.htm	
International Gynecologic Cancer Society	Yes	http://www.igcs.org/	IGCS PO Box 6387 Louisville KY 40206 USA Tel: 1 (502) 891.4575 FAX 1 (502) 891.4576
Asia Oceania Research Organization on Genital Infection and Neoplasia (AOGIN)	Asian Countries	http://www.aogin.com/pages/index.php	Email: info@aogin.com
American Radium Society	No	http://www.americanradiumsociety.org/	American Radium Society 11300 W. Olympic Blvd. Suite 600 Los Angeles, CA 90064 Phone: 310-437-0581 Ext. 123 Fax: 310-437-0585
American Society of Clinical Oncology (ASCO)	Ni	http://www.asco.org/	American Society of Clinical Oncology 1900 Duke Street, Suite 200 Alexandria, VA 22314 Tel: 703-299-0150 Fax: 703-299-1044 E-mail: asco@asco.org
American Society of Colposcopists and Cervical Pathology	No	http://www.asccp.org/	20 West Washington Street, Suite 1 Hagerstown MD 21740 Tel: (301) 733-3640 Toll Free: 1-800-787-7227 Fax (301) 733-5775

American Society for Therapeutic and Radiation oncology (ASTRO)	No	http://www.astro.org/	8280 Willow Oaks Corporate Dr. Suite 500 Fairfax VA 22031 Tel: (703) 502-1550 Toll Free: 1-800-962-7876 Fax: (703) 502-7852
European Society of Gynecologic Oncology (ESGO)	No	http://www.esgo.org/	17 Rue du Cendrier P.O. Box 1726 CH-1211 Geneva 1 Switzerland Tel: +41 22 906 9150 Fax: +41 22 732 2852 E-mail: info@esgo.org
European Society of Medical Oncology (ESMO)	No	http://www.esmo.org/	Via La Santa 7 CH-6962 Viganello Lugano Switzerland Tel: 41 (0) 91 973 19 00 FAX: 41 (0) 91 973 19 02 Email: esmo@esmo.org
European Society of Therapeutic Radiology and Oncology (ESTRO)	No	http://www.estro.be/	Avenue E. Mounierlaan 83, 1200 Brussels Tel.: +32 2 775 93 40 Fax: +32 2 779 54 94 Email: info@estro.be
International Network for Cancer Treatment and Research (INCTR)	No	http://www.inctr.org/	Institut Pasteur Rue Engeland 642 Brussels B-1180 Belgium Tel: 32(0)2-373-9323 FAX: 32-(0)2-373-9313 Email: edupont@inctr.be
International Society for Nurses in Cancer Care (ISNCC)	No	http://www.isncc.org/	108 Chestergate Macclesfield Cheshire SK11 6DU United Kingdom Tel/Fax: +44 162 566 9588 Email: secretariat@isncc.org
International Society of Gynecologic Pathology	No	http://www.isgyp.com/links.shtml	
Society of Gynecologic Oncologists (SGO)	No	http://www.sgo.org/	
Society of Gynecologic Oncology Canada	No	http://www.g-o-c.org/	780 Promenade Echo Drive Ottawa, ON K1S 5R7 Canada Tel: 613.730.4192 Ext. 250

			Tel: 1.800.561.2416 Ext. 250 Fax: 613.730.4314
Society of Pelvic Reconstructive Surgeons	No	http://www.sprs.org/	Society of Pelvic Reconstructive Surgeons 720 East 71st Street Savannah, GA 31405 Phone: 912.303.0877 Fax: 912.303.0893 Email: info@sprs.org
Others			
Open Society Oxford University Institute of Cancer medicine C-Change	No No	http://www.soros.org/ (http://www.medsci.ox.ac.uk/research/globalhealth) not the right link http://www.c-changetogether.org/default.asp	Open Society Institute 400 West 59th Street New York, NY 10019 USA Tel. 1-212-548-0600 C-Change 1776 Eye Street, N.W. Suite 900 Washington, DC 20006 Phone: (800) 830-1827 or (202) 756-1600 Fax: (202) 756-1512

SECTION 2 :
PUBLISHED RESEARCH ON CERVICAL CANCER IN THE CARIBBEAN, MEXICO AND CENTRAL AND SOUTH AMERICA

The search terms were “cervix cancer” and “control” and “program” in MEDLINE and google (760 hits: 1958-2006) 5Oct2006. Where information could be categorized, the following terms were used: Statistics (country statistics for cervical cancer incidence or mortality rates), Screening (can mean screening coverage of the population, screening test, barriers to screening, impact of screening on cervical cancer rates), Cytology (lab assessments of Pap smears), VIA (visual inspection with acetic acid), recruit (methods to recruit patients into screening), Vaccine (knowledge of the vaccine), Colp (issues related to colposcopy clinic assessments), Treatment (treatment of dysplasia or cervical cancer), Radiation (radiation therapy use in cervical cancer), and Pain (pain control), Information is categorized by country. Where an abstract was available, this was included.

Country	Area	Reference
Central and South American	Cervix cancer	*Restrepo HE. Cancer Epidemiology and control in women in Latin America and the Caribbean. PAHO 90-103* http://www.paho.org/English/DD/PUB/SP541-90-103.pdf
	Stats	GLOBCAN 2002.IARC. GLOBCAN;2002; http:/www-dep.iarc.fr/ata/T2_86403018.txt
	Stats	Sankaranarayanaan R. Cervical cancer in developing countries. Transactions of the Royal Society of Tropical medicine and Hygiene, 2002;96:580-585
	Stats	Bocciolone L, la Vecchia C, Levi F, Lucchini F, Franceschi S. Trends in uterine cancer mortality in the Americas, 1955–1988. Gynecological Oncology. 1993;51:335–344. http://www.sciencedirect.com/science?_ob=MImg&_imagekey=B6WG6-45PMTSB-9-1&_cdi=6814&_user=10843&_orig=browse&_coverDate=12%2F31%2F1993&_sk=999489996&view=c&wchp=dGLbVtb-zSkzS&md5=db1c792795ed21c919a34a915f9bd853&ie=/sdarticle.pdf Over the last two decades most Latin American countries showed declines in mortality rates ranging from about 10% in Argentina These declines were however appreciably smaller than those in the United States and Canada, where falls in uterine cancer mortality approached 50%. This diverging pattern between North and Latin America was even clearer in young women (20-44 years), when most uterine cancer originates from the cervix, and less evident in the elderly. In the young, recent upward trends were observed in Argentina.
Argentina	Stats	Regional Core Health Data Initiative, Pan American Health Organisation, 2003 14.2 new cases per 100,000 population for cervical cancer in Argentina 2000
Country	**Area**	**Reference**
Bahamas	Stats	Regional Core Health Data Initiative, Pan American Health Organisation, 2003 22.1 new cases per 100,000 population for cervical cancer in Bahamas 2000
	Coverage	No author. Cervical cancer screening in the Bahamas. Bull Pan Am Health Organ. 1996 Dec;30(4):414.
	Pain	http://www.medsch.wisc.edu/painpolicy/publicat/monograp/cmpbaha.htm Graph of Morphine consumption over time
	Pain	http://www.medsch.wisc.edu/painpolicy/publicat/monograp/cmpbarb.htm Graph of Morphine consumption over time
Barbados	Stats	Regional Core Health Data Initiative, Pan American Health Organisation, 2003 30.4 new cases per 100,000 population for cervical cancer in Barbados 2000
Belize	Stats	Regional Core Health Data Initiative, Pan American Health Organisation, 2003 39.6 new cases per 100,000 population for cervical cancer in Belize 2000

Bolivia	Recruitment Quality of Cytology	Pinto AP, Guede GB, Tuon FFB, Maia HF, Collaco LM. Cervical Cancer Screening Program of Parana: Cytohistological correlation results after 5 years. Diagn Cytopathol 2005;Oct33(4);279-83 (paper) http://www3.interscience(.wiley.com/cgi-bin/fulltext/111089060/PDFSTART
	Training	Cope – tool for setting up and evaluating a cervical screening unit developed and pilot tested in Bolivia by EngenderHealth http://www.engenderhealth.org/res/offc/qi/cope/toolbook/pdf/cope_cxca_toolbook.pdf
	Pain	http://www.medsch.wisc.edu/painpolicy/publicat/monograp/cmpboli.htm Graph of Morphine consumption over time
Brazil	Stats	Regional Core Health Data Initiative, Pan American Health Organisation, 2003 31.3 new cases per 100,000 population for cervical cancer in Brazil 2000
	Stats	Parkin et al. (eds.) Cancer Incidence in Five Continents (Vol. V, VI, VII) Malignant Neoplasm of the *Cervix uteri:*Average Annual Age-Standardized Incidence Rates (per 100,000 inhabitants, selected countries of the Americas, 1978-1992)
	Screening	Pinotti JA et al. Control of cervical cancer in Brazil. Arch AIDS Res. 1994;8(3-4):199-207. In Brazil, cervical cancer is the second most common cancer in women (20.1% of all cancers in women) after skin cancer (24.3%). It is responsible for about 5% of all cancer deaths among women in the State of Sao Paulo. The cervical cancer mortality rate does not differ among regions in Brazil, even though most health services are in metropolitan areas. In 1968, the Cervical Cancer Control Program began in Campinas. Its first phase (1968-1972) was characterized by a low number of Papanicolaou tests and a very high frequency of altered cervical cytologies. The second phase (1972-1978) was characterized by a higher number of repeat Pap tests, a high number of treatments of cervical benign lesions, and a lower frequency of altered cytologies. Geographical expansion of the program to 84 cities in the region (population of 3.5 million) characterizes the current phase, which corresponds with another increase in the frequency of altered cytologies. 85% of patients were in stages II, III, and IV before 1968 compared to only 3% after 1984. Before 1968, no one had cervical intraepithelial neoplasia while most cases (86%) had it after 1984. Therefore, the program achieved its goal of reversing the diagnosis of cervical cancer in the incurability phase to the treatable phase in the region of Campinas. In 1986, the State Health Secretariat of Sao Paulo began implementing a similar cervical cancer control program which was organized into the primary, secondary, and tertiary care levels. It increased its coverage of Pap tests from 8.38% in 1986 to about 40% in 1990. 82% of women who had undergone a consultation at Perola Byington Hospital had a Pap test during the last 2 years and almost all of these women (99%) knew that the Pap test should be repeated. Obstacles faced by the 2 programs included an increased demand in initial stages for specialized care (i.e., surgery), great exit of technicians and professionals from programs to the private sector, and inadequate follow-up of detected cases
	Screening	Zefferino C. Organization of cervical cancer screening in Campinas and surrounding region, Sao Paulo State, Brazil. Cad Saude Publica. 2006 Sep;22(9):1909-14. http://www.scielo.br/scielo.php?script=sci_arttext&pid=S0102-

		311X2006000900022&tlng=es&lng=en&nrm=iso The program was organized in a pyramid format, and the health care hierarchy was defined according to the complexity and total number of medical procedures. Screening has been extended currently to 88 municipalities, of which 51 are equipped with colposcopy and eight have facilities for treating advanced cervical cancer. The standardized incidence rate for cervical cancer in Campinas was 14.2/100,000 women per year in 1993-1995, and the standardized mortality rate per district ranged from 2.7 to 3.0 per 100,000 women in 1997-1998. This project has clearly shown that hierarchical and decentralized organization of health procedures is a necessary condition for achieving the goals of an effective cervical cancer screening program.
	Screening	de Quadros C, Victora C G, Costa J. Coverage and focus of a cervical cancer prevention program in southern Brazil. Rev Panam Salud Publica. 2004;16(4):223-32 OBJECTIVE: To determine the coverage and focus of cervical cancer screening (Pap smears) in a population-based sample in Brazil. METHODS: Cross-sectional cluster survey covering 1730 women aged 20 years or older with a history of sexual activity. Information was collected on social, demographic and behavioral variables, knowledge of and use of the Pap test. RESULTS: Of women aged 25-59 years, who are the target population of the national cervical cancer screening program, 78.7% had had at least one Pap test in their lifetime, and 68.8% had had a Pap test in the last 3 years. Statistics for focus of the program showed that of the 637 women who reported having a Pap test in the last year, only 20.6% actually required one. The remainder were either outside the age range or had had another test less than 30 months previously. Prevalence of not having been tested in the previous 3 years was highest among black (41.7%) and low-income women (64.3%), and among those at greatest risk for cervical cancer (62.3% for women with three or more risk factors). Focus was inversely related to socioeconomic status. CONCLUSION: Coverage rates were similar to those reported in other national studies, but this is the first report to examine the focus of the national program. We show that 8 of every 10 Pap tests were not necessary. Coverage levels remain unacceptably low among women of low socioeconomic status and those at greatest risk for cervical cancer.
	HPV types	Franco E, Villa L, Rohan T, Ferenzy A et al. Design and methods of the Ludwig-McGill longitudinal cohort study of the natural history of HPV infection and cervical neoplasia in Brazil. *Rev Panam Salud Pública, oct. 1999 6(4):223-33* This article reports on a large longitudinal study, begun in 1993, of the natural history of human papillomavirus (HPV) infection and cervical neoplasia in a population of low-income women in São Paulo, Brazil, a city with one of the highest risks worldwide for cervical cancer. Known as the Ludwig-McGill cohort study, the epidemiological investigation focuses on persistent infection with oncogenic HPV types as the precursor event leading to cervical neoplasia. The objectives of this study are to: 1) study the epidemiology of persistent cervical HPV infection in asymptomatic women, 2) investigate whether persistent HPV infection increases risk of low-grade and high-grade

		cervical lesions, 3) search for determinants of persistent HPV infection, 4) search for molecular variants of HPV that may be associated with an increased risk of lesions, 5) investigate whether viral burden is correlated with persistent infections and with lesion risk, 6) study the antibody response to HPV as a predictor of persistence and lesion progression, and 7) examine the role of HLA typing and codon 72 p53 gene polymorphism in mediating HPV persistence and lesion severity. The study accrued 2 528 female subjects through March 1997. Subjects were followed up every 4 months in the first year, with twice-yearly return visits to take place in subsequent years. Participants undergo a questionnaire-based interview, have a cervical specimen taken for Pap cytology and HPV testing, and have a blood sample drawn for HPV antibody testing. A cervicography is performed once in the first year and every two years thereafter. In this article we describe the design and methods of the study, provide baseline cohort characteristics, and present a preliminary assessment of the prognostic value of baseline HPV status.
	VIA	Naud P, Mator J et al. Cervical cancer Screening in Porto Alegre Brazil: Alternative methods for detecting cancer precursors in a Developing country. JLTGD 2001;5(10):24-28 OBJECTIVE: This study was conducted to test the performance characteristics of cervical cancer screening by visual inspection of the cervix with acetic acid and iodine solution. METHODS: A total of 100 women were screened for cervical cancer by Pap smear and naked eye inspection of the cervix after application of acetic acid and iodine solution. RESULTS: Comparing visual inspection to the Pap test, a sensitivity of 85.7%, specificity of 78.5%, and concordance of 79% ($p < .0011$) was established. Comparing the Pap test with colposcopy, the corresponding figures were 42.9%, 92.3%, and 66.6% ($p < .077$), respectively. Visual inspection compared to colposcopy showed corresponding figures of 100%, 7.7%, and 55.5% ($p = .48$), respectively. Colposcopy and biopsy had an agreement of 100%. CONCLUSIONS: Visual inspection with acetic acid and iodine solution proved to be a reasonable method of screening for cervical cancer precursors.
	Colp	Kalakun L, Bozzetti MC. Evolution of uterine cervical cancer mortality from 1979-1998 in the state of Rio Grande do Sul, Brazil. Cad Saude Publica, Rio de Janeiro 21(1):299-309,Jan-Fev 2005 http://www.scielo.br/scielo.php?script=sci_arttext&pid=S0102-311X2005000100033&tlng=es&lng=en&nrm=iso A decrease in uterine cervical cancer (CC) mortality has been observed in developed countries. However, mortality data in Brazil suggest that CC is one of the most frequent causes of cancer death in women; it is the fourth cause of death from cancer in women in Rio Grande Sul State. A time-trend ecological study was performed to analyze CC mortality trends in Rio Grande do Sul from 1979 to 1998. Data were collected from the Mortality Information System, Brazilian Ministry of Health (DATASUS). Standardized mortality ratios were calculated and linear regression was used for time-trend analysis. The impact of cervical cancer death on life expectancy was also estimated for the study population using potential years of life lost (PYLL). Standardized mortality ratios during the study period revealed a positive linear trend of 0.17, and the mean annual

		mortality rate was 7.58/100,000. Cervical cancer accounted for 21.9 +/- 1.33 PYLL during the period. In conclusion, although CC is a preventable and curable disease, an increase is observed in mortality from this cause in Rio Grande do Sul State, which may suggest failure in screening programs for cervical cancer
	Pain	http://www.medsch.wisc.edu/painpolicy/publicat/monograp/cmpbraz.htm Graph of Morphine consumption over time
Caribbean	Screening	Salas I. Methodology for reorganization of the cervical cancer program in Chile. Cancer Detect Prev 2006;30(1):38-43
	Cytology	Prabhaker P, Barnett B. External quality assessment of cervical baginal cytology laboratory screening in the Caribbean. West Indian Med J 1997 46 (S2):23
	Pain	http://www.medsch.wisc.edu/painpolicy/publicat/monograp/cmpchil.htm Graph of Morphine consumption over time
Chile	Stats	Regional Core Health Data Initiative, Pan American Health Organisation, 2003 29.2 new cases per 100,000 population for cervical cancer in Chile 2000
	Stats	Parkin et al. (eds.) Cancer Incidence in Five Continents (Vol. V, VI, VII) Malignant Neoplasm of the *Cervix uteri:*Average Annual Age-Standardized Incidence Rates (per 100,000 inhabitants, selected countries of the Americas, 1978-1992)
	Pain	http://www.medsch.wisc.edu/painpolicy/publicat/monograp/encachil.htm Graph of Morphine needs versus consumption
	Pain	http://www.medsch.wisc.edu/painpolicy/publicat/monograp/cmpcolo.htm Graph of Morphine consumption over time
Colombia	Stats	Parkin et al. (eds.) Cancer Incidence in Five Continents (Vol. V, VI, VII) Malignant Neoplasm of the *Cervix uteri:*Average Annual Age-Standardized Incidence Rates (per 100,000 inhabitants, selected countries of the Americas, 1978-1992)
	Screening techniques	Robles SC, Periago MR. Guanacaste, Costa Rica: a landmark for cervical cancer prevention Rev Panam Salud Publica 2004Feb15(2):73-4 (paper – editorial)
	Pain	http://www.medsch.wisc.edu/painpolicy/publicat/monograp/encacolo.htm Graph of Morphine needs versus consumption
Costa Rica	Stats	Bocciolone L, la Vecchia C, Levi F, Lucchini F, Franceschi S. Trends in uterine cancer mortality in the Americas, 1955–1988. Gynecological Oncology. 1993;51:335–344. http://www.sciencedirect.com/science?_ob=MImg&_imagekey=B6WG6-45PMTSB-9-1&_cdi=6814&_user=10843&_orig=browse&_coverDate=12%2F31%2F1993&_sk=999489996&view=c&wchp=dGLbVtb-zSkzS&md5=db1c792795ed21c919a34a915f9bd853&ie=/sdarticle.pdf Mortality rates: This diverging pattern between North and Latin America was even clearer in young women (20-44 years), when most uterine cancer originates from the cervix, and less evident in the elderly. In the young, recent upward trends were observed in Argentina, Costa Rica, and the Dominican Republic
	Stats	Parkin et al. (eds.) Cancer Incidence in Five Continents (Vol. V, VI, VII) Malignant Neoplasm of the *Cervix uteri:*Average Annual Age-Standardized Incidence Rates (per 100,000 inhabitants, selected countries of the Americas, 1978-1992)

		Herrero R et al. Determinants of geographical variations of cervical cancer in Costa Rica. Bulletin of the PAHO, 1993,27;15-25
		Sierra R et al, Cancer in Costa Rica, Lyon, IARC. 1988 Technical Report No 1
		Herrero R, Schiffman M, Bratti C, Hildescheim A, Balmaced I, Sherman ME et al Design and methods of a population-based natural history study of cervical neoplasia in a rural province of Cost Rica: the Guanacaste Project Reb Panam Salud publica 1997;1(5):362-375
		Bratti MC. Description of a sever-year prospective study of human papillomavirus infection and cervical neoplasia among 10,000 women in Guanacaster, Cost Rica. Rev Panam Salud Publica 2004;15(2):75-89
	HPV testing	Schiffman et al. HPV DNA testing in cervical cancer screening: results from women in high-risk province of Costa Rica. JAMA 2000;283, 87-93 http://jama.ama-assn.org/cgi/reprint/283/1/87 Objective To provide comprehensive data on the screening performance of HPV testing for the most common carcinogenic types, at different levels of analytic sensitivity. Design Laboratory analysis conducted during 1993-1995, using 3 cytologic techniques and cervicography, followed by colposcopic examination of women with any abnormal cervical finding, to detect all high-grade intraepithelial lesions and cancer (reference standard of clinically significant disease). The HPV testing was performed subsequently with masking regarding clinical findings. Setting Guanacaste Province, Costa Rica, a region with a high age-adjusted incidence of cervical cancer. Participants Of 11,742 randomly selected women, 8554 nonpregnant, sexually active women without hysterectomies underwent initial HPV DNA testing using the original Hybrid Capture Tube test; a stratified subsample of 1119 specimens was retested using the more analytically sensitive second generation assay, the Hybrid Capture II test. Main Outcome Measures Receiver operating characteristic analysis of detection of cervical high-grade intraepithelial lesions and cancer by HPV DNA testing based on different cut points of positivity. Results An analytic sensitivity of 1.0 pg/mL using the second generation assay would have permitted detection of 88.4% of 138 high-grade lesions and cancers (all 12 cancers were HPV-positive), with colposcopic referral of 12.3% of women. Papanicolaou testing using atypical squamous cells of undetermined significance as a cut point for referral resulted in 77.7% sensitivity and 94.2% specificity, with 6.9% referred. Specificity of the second generation assay for positivity for high-grade lesions and cancer was 89.0%, with 33.8% of remaining HPV DNA–positive subjects having low-grade or equivocal microscopically evident lesions. The higher detection threshold of 10 pg/mL used with the original assay had a sensitivity of 74.8% and a specificity of 93.4%. Lower levels of detection with the second generation assay (<1 pg/mL) proved clinically nonspecific without gains in diagnostic sensitivity. Conclusions In this study population, a cut point of 1.0 pg/mL using the second generation assay permitted sensitive detection of cervical high-grade lesions and cancer, yielding an apparently optimal trade-off between high sensitivity and reasonable specificity for this test. The test will perform best in settings in which sensitive detection of high-grade lesions and cancer is paramount. Because HPV prevalence varies by population, HPV testing positive predictive value for detection of high-grade lesions and cancer will vary accordingly, with implications for utility relative to other cervical cancer screening methods.
	HPV	Herrero R, Hildesheim A, Bratti C. Population-based study of Human

		Papillomavirus infection and cervical neoplasia in rural Costa Rica. JNCI 92(6):464-74, 2000 (Pdf article in) http://jncicancerspectrum.oxfordjournals.org/cgi/reprint/jnci;92/6/464.pdf BACKGROUND: Human papillomavirus (HPV) is the main cause of cervical neoplasia. Because few population-based studies have investigated the prevalence of type-specific infection in relation to cervical disease, we studied a high-risk population, estimating the prevalence of HPV infection and the risk associated with various HPV types. METHODS: We screened 9175 women in Guanacaste, Costa Rica, to obtain a referent standard final diagnosis, and tested 3024 women for more than 40 types of HPV with a polymerase chain reaction-based system. RESULTS: Among women with normal cytology, HPV infections peaked first in women younger than 25 years, and they peaked again at age 55 years or older with predominantly non-cancer-associated types of HPV and uncharacterized HPV types. Low-grade squamous intraepithelial lesions (LSILs) (n = 189) decreased consistently with age. The prevalence of high-grade squamous intraepithelial lesions (HSILs) (n = 128) peaked first around age 30 years and again at age 65 years or older. Seventy-three percent of LSILs were HPV positive, with HPV16 being the predominant type (16% of positive subjects). HPV was found in 89% of HSILs and 88% of cancers, with HPV16 being strongly predominant (51% and 53% of positive subjects). Virtually all HSILs and cancers had cancer-associated HPV types, with high odds ratios (ORs) and attributable fractions around 80%. Risk for HPV16 was particularly high (OR for HSILs = 320, 95% confidence interval [CI] = 97-1000; OR for cancer = 710, 95% CI = 110-4500). CONCLUSIONS: We confirm the early decline of HPV infection with age but note increased prevalence after menopause, which could be related to a second peak of HSILs, an observation that warrants further investigation. At least 80% of HPVs involved in cervical carcinogenesis in this population have been characterized. Polyvalent vaccines including the main cancer-associated HPV types may be able to prevent most cases of cervical disease in this region.
	HPV	Herrero R, Castle PE, Schiffman M. et al Epidemiologic profile of type specific human papillomavirus infection and cervical neoplasia in Guanacaste, Costa Rica. J Infect Dis. 2005;191(11):1796-807
	Pain	http://www.medsch.wisc.edu/painpolicy/publicat/monograp/cmpcost.htm Graph of Morphine consumption over time
Cuba	Stats	Regional Core Health Data Initiative, Pan American Health Organisation, 2003 23.8 new cases per 100,000 population for cervical cancer in Cuba 2000
	Stats	Bocciolone L, la Vecchia C, Levi F, Lucchini F, Franceschi S. Trends in uterine cancer mortality in the Americas, 1955–1988. Gynecological Oncology. 1993;51:335–344. http://www.sciencedirect.com/science?_ob=MImg&_imagekey=B6WG6-45PMTSB-9-1&_cdi=6814&_user=10843&_orig=browse&_coverDate=12%2F31%2F1993&_sk=999489996&view=c&wchp=dGLbVtb-zSkzS&md5=db1c792795ed21c919a34a915f9bd853&ie=/sdarticle.pdf

		There has been no fall in decline of cervix cancer in Dominican Republic This diverging pattern between North and Latin America was even clearer in young women (20-44 years), when most uterine cancer originates from the cervix, and less evident in the elderly. In the young, recent upward trends were observed in Argentina, Costa Rica, and the Dominican Republic
	Screening	Fernandez Garrotte L, Lence Ante JJ. Evaluation of the cervical cancer control program in Cuba. Bulletin of the PAHO 1996;30,387-391
	Pain	http://www.medsch.wisc.edu/painpolicy/publicat/monograp/enccuba.htm Graph of Morphine needs versus consumption
Dominica	Recruitment	Anita L. Dohn , Andrea Chávez , Michael N. Dohn , Luis Saturria , Carlos Pimentel Changes in health indicators related to health promotion and microcredit programs in the Dominican Republic JPAHO 2004;15 (3):185-93 http://journal.paho.org/?a_ID=486 Women's health (specifically cervical cancer screening). The microcredit program made small loans to individuals to start or expand small businesses. Multisector development is known to be important on a macroeconomic scale. The results of this pilot project support the view that multisector development is also important on a microeconomic level, given that the parallel microcredit and health promotion programs resulted in greater change in the measured health indicators than either program alone.
Dominican Republic	Stats	Regional Core Health Data Initiative, Pan American Health Organisation, 2003 38.4 new cases per 100,000 population for cervical cancer in Dominican Republic 2000
	Stats	Bocciolone L, la Vecchia C, Levi F, Lucchini F, Franceschi S. Trends in uterine cancer mortality in the Americas, 1955–1988. Gynecological Oncology. 1993;51:335–344. http://www.sciencedirect.com/science?_ob=MImg&_imagekey=B6WG6-45PMTSB-9-1&_cdi=6814&_user=10843&_orig=browse&_coverDate=12%2F31%2F1993&_sk=999489996&view=c&wchp=dGLbVtb-zSkzS&md5=db1c792795ed21c919a34a915f9bd853&ie=/sdarticle.pdf Over the last two decades most Latin American countries (with the exception of the Dominican Republic and Ecuador) showed declines in mortality rates ranging from about 10% in Argentina and Mexico to 25-35% in Cuba, Chile, Uruguay, and Venezuela. These declines were however appreciably smaller than those in the United States and Canada, where falls in uterine cancer mortality approached 50%. In comparison with recent rates in the United States and Canada (around 5/100,000), mortality from uterine cancer was still high in all Central and South American countries (between 11 and 20/100,000), with the sole exception of Puerto Rico (6.3/100,000). The highest rates were in Paraguay and Ecuador (over 20/100,000). The overall variation in all age-standardized uterine cancer mortality in Latin America remained around threefold during the period 1965-1988 (i.e., between 22/100,000 in Paraguay and 6.3/100,000 in Puerto Rico). However, if the United States and Canada were also considered, the ratio between the highest and lowest mortality rate at all ages increased from about threefold during the period 1965-1969 to over fourfold in the late 1980s. This diverging pattern between North and Latin America was

		even clearer in young women (20-44 years), when most uterine cancer originates from the cervix, and less evident in the elderly. In the young, recent upward trends were observed in Argentina, Costa Rica, and the Dominican Republic.
	Pain	http://www.medsch.wisc.edu/painpolicy/publicat/monograp/cmpecua.htm Graph of Morphine consumption over time
Ecuador	Stats	Regional Core Health Data Initiative, Pan American Health Organisation, 2003 44.2 new cases per 100,000 population for cervical cancer in Ecuador 2000
	Recruit	Aguito I, Bishop A. Perceived barriers and benefits of cervical cancer screening in Latin America. Preventive Medicine 2004;49:91-8 http://www.sciencedirect.com/science?_ob=MImg&_imagekey=B6WPG-4CCF94C-2-1&_cdi=6990&_user=10843&_orig=browse&_coverDate=07%2F31%2F2004&_sk=999609998&view=c&wchp=dGLbVzz-zSkWW&md5=ff06818626496f2eeeebbd037e0db590&ie=/sdarticle.pdf Except for the accessibility and availability of quality services, these results are consistent with findings from other studies in developed and developing countries. Barriers could be lifted if health service delivery was enhanced, for instance, through quality improvement techniques that are available at low cost. Women's anxiety over test results still needs to be further assessed to devise risk communication strategies that take into account broader cultural frameworks. It is to be noted that such strategies should permeate the way health services are provided for cervical cancer prevention regardless of the specific test used. Vulnerability perceived by low-income women with respect to their capacity to cope with diseases and trust the health services and how this affects their perceptions of risk and their behaviors have not been studied as yet.
	Screening	Aguto I, Sandoval J et al. Improving cervical cancer prevention in a developing country. Int J Quality in Health Care 18(2):2006, 81-86 http://ncd.bvsalud.org/portals/cervicalCancer/docs/en/dossier_Cabanas.doc (PAHO project description) http://intqhc.oxfordjournals.org/cgi/reprint/mzi100?ijkey=zD1Dz1p9ej2rozI&keytype=ref Showed that they could improve screening of the priority population according to guidelines (3408 new first time screenings in middle age group), improve test taking (fall in unsatisfactory tests by 50%), reduce turn around time (fall by 1/3) and improve followup rates (by 24%)
	Issues	http://www.path.org/files/RH_cryo_white_paper.pdf Problems to access treatment: cost of transportation, looking for ways through the ministry of health to support transport of patients to San Salvador All cancer treatment is paid for by the Ministry of Health or by private donations to Instituto del Cancer
El Salvador	Stats	Regional Core Health Data Initiative, Pan American Health Organisation, 2003 40.6 new cases per 100,000 population for cervical cancer in El Salvador 2000
	Pain	http://www.medsch.wisc.edu/painpolicy/publicat/monograp/cmpelsa.htm

		Graph of Morphine consumption over time
French Guiana	Stats	1998 Health Report P271, http://www.paho.org/english/HIA1998/FrenchGuiana.pdf Describes number of hospitals and other resources
	Stats	Regional Core Health Data Initiative, Pan American Health Organisation, 2003 51.1 new cases per 100,000 population for cervical cancer in Guyana 2000
Grenada	Stats	Regional Core Health Data Initiative, Pan American Health Organisation, 2003 93.9 new cases per 100,000 population for cervical cancer in Haiti 2000
	Pain	http://www.medsch.wisc.edu/painpolicy/publicat/monograp/cmphait.htm Graph of Morphine consumption over time
	Pain	www.med.unc.edu/hha/Cervical-Cancer-Prevention-Strategies.pdf More of a review of the literature with some local context
Guatemala	Stats	Regional Core Health Data Initiative, Pan American Health Organisation, 2003 39.6 new cases per 100,000 population for cervical cancer in Guatemala 2000
	Screening	http://ncd.bvsalud.org/portals/cervicalCancer/docs/en/GuatemalaCC.doc 2002 by PAHO Subsequent to the needs assessment, the Guatemalan Working Group designed a pilot project to organize a screening and treatment program in 5 health districts which would actively recruit women aged 25-59 years of age for screening and referral to diagnosis and treatment, if indicated
	Pain	http://www.medsch.wisc.edu/painpolicy/publicat/monograp/cmpguat.htm Graph of Morphine consumption over time
Guyana	Stats	www.who.int/countries/en/cooperation_strategy_ven_en.pdf Pg 10
	Stats	Regional Core Health Data Initiative, Pan American Health Organisation, 2003 51.1 new cases per 100,000 population for cervical cancer in Guyana 2000
Haiti	Stats	Regional Core Health Data Initiative, Pan American Health Organisation, 2003 93.9 new cases per 100,000 population for cervical cancer in Haiti 2000
	Pain	http://www.medsch.wisc.edu/painpolicy/publicat/monograp/cmphait.htm Graph of Morphine consumption over time
Honduras	Stats	Regional Core Health Data Initiative, Pan American Health Organisation, 2003 39.6 new cases per 100,000 population for cervical cancer in Honduras 2000
	Screening	http://www.medsch.wisc.edu/painpolicy/publicat/monograp/cmpjama.htm Graph of Morphine consumption over time
	Pain	http://www.medsch.wisc.edu/painpolicy/publicat/monograp/cmphond.htm Graph of Morphine consumption over time
Jamaica	Stats	Hoyo C, Miller WC, Newman BM et al. Selective screening for cervical neoplasia: an approach for resource-poor settings. Int J Epidemiol. 2000 Oct;29(5):807-12. http://ije.oxfordjournals.org/cgi/reprint/29/5/807

		To screen selectively, we developed two risk scores using data from a population-based case-control study in Jamaica with 202 cases and 363 controls. Independent risk factors for cervical neoplasia were determined using logistic regression. An unweighted risk score for each subject was developed by a simple count of risk factors present and a weighted risk score was calculated by summing regression coefficients for each risk factor. RESULTS: Four patient characteristics were independently predictive of cervical neoplasia, older age (OR = 3.4, 95% CI : 1.8-6.7), > or = 4 pregnancies (OR = 5.6, 95% CI : 1.2-18.7), poverty (OR = 2.1, 95% CI : 1.3-3.3) and cigarette smoking (OR = 1.9, 95% CI : 1.2-3.2). Using cut-off points of > or = 20 for the weighted scores and > 3 for unweighted scores, the sensitivity and specificity were 65% and 69% for the unweighted score and 75% and 61%, respectively, for the weighted score. Areas under the receiver operating characteristic (ROC) curves for the weighted versus the unweighted scores were similar, suggesting similar overall accuracy. CONCLUSION: Selective screening using risk assessment strategies is potentially useful, particularly in resource-poor settings. However, whether weighting factors is essential is dependent on prevalence of factors in a given setting. Although this approach needs validation in other populations, women at highest risk for cervical neoplasia can be identified using demographic factors available during a regular clinic visit.
	Recruit	Regional Core Health Data Initiative, Pan American Health Organisation, 2003 43.4 new cases per 100,000 population for cervical cancer in Jamaica 2000
	Pain	http://www.medsch.wisc.edu/painpolicy/publicat/monograp/cmpjama.htm Graph of Morphine consumption over time
Martinique	Stats	Parkin et al. (eds.) Cancer Incidence in Five Continents (Vol. V, VI, VII) Malignant Neoplasm of the *Cervix uteri:* Average Annual Age-Standardized Incidence Rates (per 100,000 inhabitants, selected countries of the Americas, 1978-1992)
Mexico	Stats	Bocciolone L, la Vecchia C, Levi F, Lucchini F, Franceschi S. Trends in uterine cancer mortality in the Americas, 1955–1988. Gynecological Oncology. 1993;51:335–344. http://www.sciencedirect.com/science?_ob=MImg&_imagekey=B6WG6-45PMTSB-9-1&_cdi=6814&_user=10843&_orig=browse&_coverDate=12%2F31%2F1993&_sk=999489996&view=c&wchp=dGLbVtb-zSkzS&md5=db1c792795ed21c919a34a915f9bd853&ie=/sdarticle.pdf Over the last two decades most Latin American countries showed declines in mortality rates ranging from about 10% in Mexico
	Stats	Regional Core Health Data Initiative, Pan American Health Organisation, 2003 40.5 new cases per 100,000 population for cervical cancer in Mexico 2000
	Stats	Palacio-Mejja LS, Rangel-Gomez G et al. Cervical cancer, a disease of poverty: mortality differences between urban and rural areas in Mexico. Salud Publica Mex. 2003;45 Suppl 3:S315-25. http://www.insp.mx/salud/index.html. OBJECTIVE: To examine cervical cancer mortality rates in Mexican urban and rural communities, and their association with poverty-related factors, during 1990-2000. MATERIAL AND METHODS: We analyzed data from national databases to obtain mortality trends and regional variations using a

		Poisson regression model based on location (urban-rural). RESULTS: During 1990-2000 a total of 48,761 cervical cancer (CC) deaths were reported in Mexico (1990 = 4,280 deaths/year; 2000 = 4,620 deaths/year). On average, 12 women died every 24 hours, with 0.76% yearly annual growth in CC deaths. Women living in rural areas had 3.07 higher CC mortality risks compared to women with urban residence. Comparison of state CC mortality rates (reference = Mexico City) found higher risk in states with lower socio-economic development (Chiapas, relative risk [RR] = 10.99; Nayarit, RR = 10.5). Predominantly rural states had higher CC mortality rates compared to Mexico City (lowest rural population). CONCLUSIONS: CC mortality is associated with poverty-related factors, including lack of formal education, unemployment, low socio-economic level, rural residence and insufficient access to healthcare. This indicates the need for eradication of regional differences in cancer detection.
	Know-ledge	Lazcano-Ponce E, Rivera L, Arillo-Santillan E et al. Acceptability of a human papillomavirus (HPV) trial vaccine among mothers of adolescents in Cuernavaca, Mexico. Arch Med Res 2001;32(3);243-7 Acceptability of partents – 84%. 80% of women with daughters 10-15 yo. Correlates of acceptability – knowledge of benefits of HPV vaccine and history of 2 or more sexual partners
	Recruit	Torres-Mejia G, Salmeron-Castro J et al.Characteristics of respondents to a cervical cancer screening program in a developing country. Arch Med Res. 2002 May-Jun;33(3):295-300. BACKGROUND: Characteristics associated with the response to a personalized, mailed invitation for the Papanicolaou (Pap) test vary among women. This study assesses the relationship between selected characteristics (e.g., demographic, obstetric, Pap history) and the response to a letter of invitation to undergo a Pap test among Mexican women affiliated with the Mexican Social Security Institute (IMSS). METHODS: Study subjects were 328 women affiliated with the IMSS who received and responded to a mailed letter of invitation, and 247 age- and clinically matched controls who received but did not respond to the letter of invitation. Statistical analysis consisted of multivariate conditional regression model. RESULTS: Having better housing conditions was one of the factors associated with letter response (medium level vs. low level, odds ratio [OR] = 3.17, 95% confidence interval [95% CI] = 2.46-4.09; high level vs. low level, OR = 2.65, 95% CI = 2.06-3.41). Other factors positively associated with letter response were greater number of pregnancies, previous Pap testing, being pleased at receipt of the letter of invitation, and knowing another woman who had received the invitation. Factors associated negatively to letter response were 7 or more years of formal education (> or =7 years vs. 0-6 years, OR = 0.50, 95% CI = 0.40-0.63), having a current job, availability of other medical services in addition to the IMSS, and willingness to receive Pap results by mail. CONCLUSIONS: Low educational level is not a limitation for cervical cancer screening call and recall among women affiliated with the IMSS.
	Recruit	Lazcano-ponce EC, Moss S et al. The factors that determine participation in cervical cancer screening in the state of Morelos. Salud Publica Mex. 1999 Jul-Aug;41(4):278-85 OBJECTIVE: To determine the main factors associated to participation in an early detection program of cancer (DPC), in a population with a high

		cervical cancer (CC) mortality rate. MATERIAL AND METHODS: A population-based, cross-sectional study was performed in the state of Morelos, which included 3,197 women aged between 15 and 49 years, randomly selected from a household sample frame of the 33 municipalities of the state. RESULTS: Awareness of the utility of the Papanicolaou (Pap) test (OR 29.6, 95% CI 23.6-37) and a former history of gynecological symptoms (OR 1.7, 95% CI 1.2-2.4) predisposed to greater use of the DPC. Factors associated to the use of the Pap test were precedents of using one contraceptive (OR 1.4, 95% CI 1.1-1.8) or two or more contraceptives (OR 2.1, 95% CI 1.6-2.8). CONCLUSIONS: In the state of Morelos, Mexico, screening for cervical cancer is offered opportunistically in the context of health care use. Therefore, the precedent of using health care services is the main determining factor for use of the DPC program. These results reveal the need to design alternative strategies to promote participation among women who have no access to health services, since they constitute the population group at highest risk of developing CC.
	Recruit	Torres-Mejia G, Salmeron-castro J et al. Call and recall for cervical cancer screening in a developing country: a randomised field trial. Int J Cancer. 2000 Sep 15;87(6):869-73. http://www3.interscience.wiley.com/cgi-bin/fulltext/72516358/PDFSTART A randomised field trial was used to assess Mexican women's response to a mailed invitation for a Papanicolaou test. A sample of 4,802 women, 20 to 64 years old, chosen at random from the Mexican Social Security Institute Register were randomly assigned to an intervention and to a control group. A letter of invitation and a reminder were sent to the intervention group. A letter was also sent to the control group at the end of the follow-up period (8.5 weeks) in order to compare the response among women who received a letter in both groups. Cumulative incidence and incidence rates were used to determine the response and the speed of response, respectively. The response among women who had received the letter was 33.5% (efficacy) in the intervention group, while 5.9% ($p<0.001$) in the control group attended a Papanicolaou test. For the total of women invited, the response was 20.1% (effectiveness) and 3.3% ($p<0.001$), respectively. The response was greater in rural areas (rural vs. urban/suburban; $p = 0.002$) and eldest women (50-64 vs. 20-49; p = 0. 02). The response rate was 7 times grater in the intervention than in the control group (RR = 7.1; 95% CI 5.4-9.4; $p < 0.001$). A mailed invitation to have a Papanicolaou test substantially increases attendance by women who receive it. A mailed reminder improves results. This strategy could be implemented in addition to the ones already in use, mainly among rural and elderly women. Copyright 2000 Wiley-Liss, Inc.
	Screening	Aquilar-Perez JA, Levva-Lopez AG et al. Cervical cancer screening: knowledge of Pap smear benefits and utilization in Mexico. Rev Saude Publica. 2003 Feb;37(1):100-6. http://www.scielo.br/scielo.php?script=sci_arttext&pid=S0034-89102003000100015&tlng=en&lng=en&nrm=iso OBJECTIVE: To identify and evaluate the predisposing factors regarding the utilization of the Pap smears in the population seen in the Cervical Cancer Screening Program in Mexico METHODS: A cross-sectional study was conducted from January 1997 through December 1998 in Mexico city.

		A questionnaire was applied to a total of 2,107 women of reproductive age who attended a family planning program and data was collected regarding the following topics: social-demographics, reproductive risk factors associated with cervical cancer, sexual behavior and partner history, birth control, knowledge about Pap smear' benefits, and its utilization. Statistic analysis was conducted using Student' s test and non-conditional multiple logistic regression model for determining significance. RESULTS: The predisposing factors were: knowledge about Pap smear's benefits (OR=6.00, CI 95% 4.70-7.67), history of using at least two birth control methods (OR=2.38, CI 95% 1.75-3.24), previous history of vaginal infection (OR=2.18, CI 95% 1.73-2.75), sexual partner's approval of gynecological examinations (OR=1.56, CI 95% 1.07-2.29). CONCLUSIONS: Educational programs on cancer prevention in this population should include the benefits of screening tests. Pap smears for Mexican women of reproductive age are mostly offered opportunely. The previous use of health services is a determinant factor for the utilization of the Cervical Cancer Screening Program. These results show the need to strengthen health promotion programs to women at high risk of cervical cancer and their sexual partners.
	Screening	Lazcano-Ponce EC, Moss S et al. The positive experience of screening quality among users of a cervical cancer detection center.Arch Med Res. 2002 Mar-Apr;33(2):186-92. BACKGROUND: Our objective was to determine the main factors associated with increased utilization of a cervical cancer screening program (CCSP) in a population with a high mortality rate due to cervical cancer. METHODS: A population-based study was carried out in the Mexican state of Morelos, Mexico. The study population included 3,197 women between the ages of 15 and 49 years who were selected at random using a State Household Sampling Framework in the State of Morelos's 33 municipalities. The sample included 2,094 women with a history of a previous Papanicolaou (Pap) test. RESULTS: A previous experience of good screening quality is strongly associated with greater use of the CCSP (OR = 4.2; 95% confidence interval [CI], 1.6-10.9). The educational level of the head of the family is related to more frequent use of Pap smear services. Women whose husbands have 13 or more years of education (OR = 1.8; 95% CI 1.1-2.9) were more likely to have been screened. Similarly, women who had used two or more family planning methods (OR = 1.6; 95% CI 1.2-2.1) and those who knew why the Pap test was given (OR = 3.0; 95% CI 2.1-4.3) had a better history of Pap screening. CONCLUSIONS: In areas where coverage of cervical cancer screening is low, a CCSP that guarantees the quality of all the different elements of care is essential if obstacles to cervical cancer prevention are to be eliminated. It is of particular importance to take into account and satisfy the perceptions and expectations of the women at risk.
	Screening	Aguito I, Bishop A. Perceived barriers and benefits of cervical cancer screening in Latin America. Preventive Medicine 2004;49:91-8 http://www.sciencedirect.com/science?_ob=MImg&_imagekey=B6WPG-4CCF94C-2-1&_cdi=6990&_user=10843&_orig=browse&_coverDate=07%2F31%2F2004&_sk=999609998&view=c&wchp=dGLbVzz-zSkWW&md5=ff06818626496f2eeeebbd037e0db590&ie=/sdarticle.pdf Except for the accessibility and availability of quality services, these results

		are consistent with findings from other studies in developed and developing countries. Barriers could be lifted if health service delivery was enhanced, for instance, through quality improvement techniques that are available at low cost. Women's anxiety over test results still needs to be further assessed to devise risk communication strategies that take into account broader cultural frameworks. It is to be noted that such strategies should permeate the way health services are provided for cervical cancer prevention regardless of the specific test used. Vulnerability perceived by low-income women with respect to their capacity to cope with diseases and trust the health services and how this affects their perceptions of risk and their behaviors have not been studied as yet.
	Screening	Najera AP, Lazcano-ponce EC, et al Factors associated with Mexican women's familiarity with the purpose of the Pap test. Bull Pan Am Health Organ. 1996 Dec;30(4):348-53. Use of health services is usually associated with a variety of factors, including the socioeconomic characteristics of the users, their familiarity with the usefulness of the services provided, and the acceptability and accessibility of those services. To study the factors associated with women's familiarity with the Pap test, a population-based study was carried out in Mexico City and two rural areas in the state of Oaxaca by means of household interviews. The sample consisted of 4208 women 15 to 49 years of age. Univariate, bivariate, and multivariate analyses were done using unconditional logistic regression; the independent variables were access to social security health services, age, education, housing quality, and place of residence (urban or rural); the dependent variable was the interview subject's familiarity with the purpose of the Pap test. The results were expressed as odds ratios with 95% confidence intervals. It was found that 41.5% of the women surveyed did not know the purpose of the Pap test, and that within this latter group, 97% had never had one. Factors found to be associated with not knowing the test's purpose were lack of access to the social security health services (OR = 1.9; 95% CI: 1.5-2.3); illiteracy (OR = 36.1; 95% CI: 17.9-72.7); and low socioeconomic level (OR = 2.9; 95% CI: 2.3-3.7). Also, rural dwellers had less familiarity with the Pap test than urban dwellers (OR = 0.5; 95% CI: 0.4-0.7). These results highlight the need to develop strategies for making the benefits of the Pap test known, bearing in mind the socioeconomic and cultural diversity of the populations involved.
	Screening	Arillo-Santillan E, Nigenda G et al. Mexico City physicians' awareness about cervical cancer prevention: implications for cancer screening. J Cancer Educ. 2001 Summer;16(2):75-9 BACKGROUND: In spite of an early cancer detection program (CCSP), Mexico has a mortality rate for cervical cancer of 16.5 per 100,000 women. METHOD: A cross-sectional study of 330 physicians at the Mexico City General Hospital evaluated their knowledge of the CCSP, etiology, diagnostic alternatives, and treatment guidelines. Variance analysis was the statistical procedure used. Replies to a questionnaire about cervical cancer prevention awareness were scored on a scale from 1 to 9. RESULTS: According to the awareness scale, the global average classification was 4.4, with 50% of the physicians scoring 4 or less. There was no difference in the CCSP knowledge scores of gynecologists (mean 4.92, 95% CI 4.2-5.3), oncologists (mean 4.85, 95% CI 4.3-5.5), pathologists (mean 5.23, 95% CI

		4.9-5.6), and those in other specialties (mean 4.29, 95% CI 4.2-5.0), p > 0.05. Many respondents attributed CCSP's lack of effectiveness to public apathy (68.12%). CONCLUSIONS: The effectiveness of the CCSP can be improved by educating health professionals if this education is combined with elimination of obstacles to its use. More information is needed to justify revising how doctors are educated in terms of not only quality of the training but also the contents of pre- and postgraduate training programs.
	Screening	Salmeron J, Lazcano-Ponce E et al. Comparison of HPV-based assays with Papanicolaou smears for cervical cancer screening in Morelos State, Mexico.Cancer Causes Control. 2003 Aug;14(6):505-12 OBJECTIVE: To compare the performance of human papillomavirus (HPV) assays with conventional Pap cytology for cervical cancer (CC) screening in Mexico. METHODS: Pap smears, self-collected vaginal specimens (SS) for HPV testing, and clinician-collected cervical specimens (CS) for HPV testing were obtained from 7868 women, aged 15-85 years old, attending CC screening at the Mexican Institute of Social Security (IMSS) between May and October, 1999. SS and CS specimens were screened for oncogenic HPV DNA by Hybrid Capture 2. Women who received cytological interpretations of atypical squamous cells of undetermined significance (ASCUS), and/or a positive HPV test were referred for colposcopy and histologic studies. The relative estimates for sensitivity, specificity and predictive values of each test were calculated using histological diagnoses of cervical intraepithelial neoplasia (CIN) grades 2 or 3, or CC histological diagnosis. RESULTS: Oncogenic HPV detection rate was 11.6% for SS, and 9.3% for CS. Pap smear abnormalities were observed in 2.4% of the women. Of 1147 women who had at least one abnormal test result, 88.5% underwent colposcopy, and 101 biopsy-confirmed CIN2/3 or cancer cases were identified. The relative sensitivity estimates for the Pap test, SS and CS were 59.4% (95% CI: 49.2-68.9), 71.3% (95% CI: 61.3-79.6), and 93.1% (95% CI: 85.8-96.9), respectively, while the specificities were 98.3% (95% CI: 98.0-98.6), 89.2% (95% CI: 88.5-89.9), and 91.8% (95% CI: 91.2-92.4), respectively. The positive predictive values of Pap, SS and CS were 36.1, 9.1 and 14.9, the colposcopy referrals needed to detect a case of CIN2/3 or cancer were 2.8, 11.0 and 6.7, respectively. DISCUSSION: Both HPV assays detected more cases of CIN2/3 or CC than Pap cytology alone. However, the HPV assays increased the number of colposcopy referrals. Our study suggests that HPV testing could be an effective way to improve the performance of CC screening.
	Screening	Lazcano-ponce EC, Aguilar PN, Alonso De Ruiz P. programa de deteccion Oportuna de cancer Cervical en mexico. 1. Diagnostico situacional. Cancerologia 42(3):123-140, Julio-Septembre 1996
	Cytology	De Ruiz PA, Lazcano-ponce EC et al. Diagnostic reproducibility of Pap testing in two regions of Mexico: the need for quality control mechanisms. Bull Pan Am Health Organ. 1996 Dec;30(4):330-8 To assess the reproducibility of diagnostic results obtained by examining Pap smears for cervical neoplasia, a study was conducted using a single group of 20 Pap smears, 3 negative and 17 from patients with varying degrees of neoplasia. These smears were examined by 14 volunteer readers (13 cytotechnologists and 1 cytopathologist) from the Mexican states of Oaxaca and Veracruz, and also by a highly experienced cytopathologist certified by the Mexican Board of Pathological Anatomy whose work

		provided a reference standard. Individual variability, as assessed by the Kappa coefficient of concordance, showed considerable difference in the diagnostic results obtained by different readers-the degree of agreement depending on the type of cervical lesion involved and the number of specimens from patients with that type of lesion. There was little diagnostic agreement when the specimens were assessed for particular classes of cervical neoplasia-mild, moderate, or severe neoplasia, carcinoma in situ, or invasive cervical cancer. (The greatest concordance was found in diagnosing specimens from subjects with invasive cervical cancer.) However, when the diagnosis was assessed continuously, using Kappa weighted in accordance with the five possible diagnoses of cervical neoplasia, the apparent reproducibility of the diagnoses improved greatly, Kappa coefficients for the 14 readers ranging from 0.31 to 0.72. In general, these data support the view that there is a need in Mexico and other parts of the Americas to establish quality control mechanisms monitoring cytologic diagnosis of cervical neoplasia, to standardize diagnostic nomenclature using a system such as the Bethesda System, to institute periodic certification, and to provide continuing training. As this suggests, it is necessary not only to evaluate but also to bring about organizational changes in order to expeditiously prevent or correct the problems that currently constrain achievement of efficient and effective cytologic diagnosis.
	Cytology	Lazcano-ponce EC, Najera-Aguilar P, Buiatti E et al. The cervical cancer screening program in Mexico: problems with access and coverage. Cancer Causes Control 8(5):698-704 Sept 1997 A cross-sectional study was carried out in two geographic regions of Mexico - Oaxaca (rural area) and Mexico City (urban area) - to determine the main factors for predicting participation in Cervical Cytology Screening Programs (CCSP), in populations with high mortality due to cervical cancer. We included 4,208 women aged between 15 and 49 years, randomly selected through a national household-sample frame. Knowledge of what the Pap test is used for strongly predisposes use of CCSP in Mexico City (odds ratio [OR] = 46.1, 95 percent confidence interval [CI] = 33.1-64.1) and Oaxaca state (OR = 61.5, CI = 42.0-89.9), as well as high socioeconomic level (Mexico: OR = 2.0, CI = 1.1-7.6; Oaxaca: OR = 4.1, CI = 3.1-5.3), high education level (Mexico: OR = 3.6, CI = 1.5-8.8; Oaxaca: OR = 5.3, CI = 2.8-10.0), and access to social security (Mexico: OR = 1.7, CI = 1.4-2.2; Oaxaca: OR = 2.2, CI = 1.8-2.7). Low coverage of the CCSP is confirmed as an important problem in Mexico.
	HPV testing vs cytology	Hernandez avila M, Lazcano-ponce EC et al Evaluation of a program for the early detection of cancer of the uterine cervix in Mexico City. A populational-based epidemiologic study of cases and controls. Gac Med Mex. 1994 Jul-Aug;130(4):201-9. Cervical cancer is still an important public health problem in Mexico; in spite of the development of various programs aimed at lowering mortality due to this disease, impact has not yet been achieved. In this study we present an evaluation of the Early Detection Program for Cervical Cancer in Mexico City. The authors carried out a case-control study with a populational base, in which a sample of cases obtained in eight hospitals and a sample of controls representative of the general population were included. We report a protective effect attributed to the program. The

		women with complete cytology showed 2.4 times less risk of cervical cancer. Nevertheless the effect of the program at a populational level is still limited because it covers only 20 per cent of the cases in the population. The results indicate the need for developing operative research programs in order to increase the demand for and the quality and efficiency of preventive services.
	Screening	Lazcano-Ponce EC et al. Cervical cancer screening in developing countries: Why is it ineffective? The case of Mexico. Archives of medical Research 1999;30;240-250 http://www.sciencedirect.com/science?_ob=MImg&_imagekey=B6VNM-3WY3Y3R-D-5&_cdi=6182&_user=10843&_orig=browse&_coverDate=05%2F06%2F1999&_sk=999699996&view=c&wchp=dGLzVlz-zSkzk&md5=474e9fb31b764b443bb84e3129c32574&ie=/sdarticle.pdf BACKGROUND: Mexico established a national cervical cancer-screening program in 1974. Despite the implementation of the program, there was a steady mortality trend of 16 per 100,000 women over 15 years. METHODS: A diagnostic procedure of the pitfalls was applied to the following steps of the screening procedure: Pap sampling quality; cytological diagnosis validity; compliance of women; and determinants of non-participation. RESULTS: The low effectiveness of screening on cervical cancer is principally due to factors associated with quality and coverage. Pap quality is deficient; 64% of a random sample of specimens lacked endocervical cells. Reading centers presented false negative indices of between 10 and 54%. Women seek screening in a late stage of disease (55% with cervical cancer seek care because they have symptoms). In addition, coverage is low; in women between 15 and 49 years of age in Mexico City, 64.2% have a history of Pap, compared with 30% in rural areas. Knowledge of what the Pap is used for strongly determines the use of screening. In rural areas, only 40% of women are informed about the purpose of the Pap test. CONCLUSIONS: A proposal to reorganize Mexico's screening program includes the following five main strategies: (a) increased coverage; (b) improved quality control of how cervical smears are taken; (c) better interpretation of Pap tests; (d) guaranteed treatment for those whose tests show abnormalities, and (e) improved follow-up
	Screening	Lazcano-Ponce EC et al. Evaluation model of the Mexican national program for early cervical cancer detection and proposals for a new approach. Cancer Causes Control, 1998, 9:241-251 An evaluation model on cervical cancer (CC) prevention in Mexico was carried out during 1990-95, using three observation units: women at risk, screening providers, and use of health services. Methods: A diagnostic procedure of the pitfalls was applied to the following steps of the screening procedure: Pap sampling quality, cytological diagnosis validity, compliance of women, and determinants of nonparticipation. Results: The low effectiveness of screening for CC is due principally to factors associated with quality and coverage. Quality of Pap is deficient; 64 percent of a random sample of specimens lacked endocervical cells. Reading centers presented false negative indices between 10 and 54 percent. Women seek screening in a late stage of disease (55 percent with CC seek

		care because they have symptoms). In addition, coverage is low; in women between 15 and 49 years of age in Mexico City, 64.2 percent have a history of Pap smears, compared with 30 percent in rural areas. Knowledge of what the Pap is used for strongly determines use of screening. In rural areas, only 40 percent know the purpose of the Pap. Conclusions: This information justifies an intervention to reorganize CC screening in Mexico, through strategies for improving compliance, quality, follow-up, and treatment for abnormal screens.
	Screening	Flisser A, Garcia-Malo F, Canepa Mde L, et al. Implementation and evaluation of an national external quality control program for cervical cytology in Mexico. Salud Publica Mex 2002 Sep-Oct 44(5):431-6
	Screening	Lazcano Ponce E, de Ruiz PA et al. Cervical cancer: new perspectives for diagnosis, prevention and control in developing countries. Salud Publica Mex. 2003;45 Suppl 3:S304-5.
	Screening	Lazcano-Ponce EC. Mortality from cervical carcinoma in Mexico: impact of screening 1980-1990 Acta Cytologica, 1996,40;506-512 OBJECTIVE: To determine the temporal mortality trends of uterine cervical cancer in Mexico for the period 1980-1990. STUDY DESIGN: In Mexico, data from death certificates are collected in a national repository at the National Institute of Statistics, Geography and Informatics. These data were analyzed to obtain mortality trends, and regional variations were obtained for the same period using a Poisson regression model. RESULTS: The official mortality figure for cervical cancer for the study period was 37,982 cases. Subregistration due to misclassification was evident, particularly in the first five years of the study period; however, poor quality of information was proportionally distributed across the different age groups. A standardized analysis by quinquennia showed a steady mortality trend during the last 10 years, with slightly upward significant trends within some age groups (beta=0, P<.05). High regional variations in cervical cancer mortality risks were found using a Poisson regression model. Twenty-four states in Mexico showed an increased mortality risk when compared with Mexico City; seven states showed a steady or downward trend. CONCLUSION: The results show the ineffectiveness of the cancer screening program, underscoring the need to ensure access to and the quality of the cervical cancer screening program in order to decrease mortality rates.
	Screening	Lazcano-Ponce, E., Evaluation model of the Mexican national program for early cervical cancer detection and proposals for a new approach. Cancer Causes Control. 1998 May;9(3):241-51.
	Screening	Salinas-Martinez AM et al. Quality of the Early Cervical Cancer Detection Program in the State of Nuevo Leon. Salud Publica Mex. 1997 May-Jun;39(3):187-94.
	Screening	Hernández-Avila M, Lazcano-Ponce EC, de Ruiz PA, Romieu I. Evaluation of the cervical cancer screening programme in Mexico: A population-based case-control study. Int J Epidemiol 1998;27:370-376. (pdf Article) http://ije.oxfordjournals.org/cgi/reprint/27/3/370 BACKGROUND: This study presents the evaluation of the Mexico City Cervical Cancer Screening Programme (CCSP). Uterine cervical cancer (CC) is still a major public health problem in Mexico. Various actions aimed at reducing mortality from CC have been unsuccessful with an

		estimated 62000 deaths reported between 1980 and 1995. METHODS: The authors performed a study of cases and controls chosen on a population basis that included a sample of 233 cases of cancer in situ, and 397 cases of invasive cervical cancer obtained from eight hospitals, and a sample of 1005 controls representative of the general population. The results are presented stratified by case type, classified according to whether the cancer is invasive or not. RESULTS: The results show low impact of the cervical cancer screening programme in Mexico. Women who had a history of use of the Papanicolaou smear (PAP), who did not seek testing due to gynaecological symptoms and who had received their PAP results, had a 2.63 times lower risk of developing invasive cervical cancer (OR = 0.38; 95% CI: 0.28-0.52). CONCLUSIONS: The principal findings of this study in relation to the low impact of the screening programme in Mexico, are the low level of existing coverage and late use of health services by women at risk.
	Screening	Hernandez-Avila M. Evaluation of a program for the early detection of cancer of the uterine cervix in Mexico City. A populational-based epidemiologic study of cases and controls. Gac Med Mex. 1994 Jul-Aug;130(4):201-9.
	Screening	Lazcano-Ponce EC, Castro R. et al. Barriers to early detection of cervical-uterine cancer in Mexico. J Womens Health. 1999 Apr;8(3):399-408 In Mexico, a woman dies of cervical-uterine cancer every 2 hours, indicating a low impact by the national program for early detection of this cancer, principally because of problems related to quality and coverage. Through a qualitative study, we identified the principal barriers to use of the detection program from the point of view of actual and potential program users. Four focus groups were organized in standard conditions in Mexico City (urban, developed) and in the southern state of Oaxaca (rural, economically disadvantaged area). Participants were either women with at least one previous Papanicolaou (Pap) test or women who had never had the test. Barriers to Pap test use included (1) lack of knowledge about cervical-uterine cancer etiology, (2) not knowing that the Pap test exists, (3) the conception that cancer is an inevitably fatal disease, (4) problems in doctor/medical institution-patient relationships, (5) giving priority to unmet needs related to extreme poverty, (6) opposition by the male sexual partner, (7) rejection of the pelvic examination, (8) long waits for sample collection and receiving results, and (9) perceived high costs for care. To increase coverage of the early detection program for cervical-uterine cancer in Mexico, the needs, perceptions, and beliefs of women and their partners must be taken into account when developing policy and planning, given the role these factors play in the decision-making process that leads to their participation or nonparticipation in this program.
	Cytology	Lazcano-Ponce EC et Al. Validity and reproducibility of cytologic diagnosis in a sample of cervical cancer screening centers in mexico. Acta Cytologica 1997;41;277-284 OBJECTIVE: To evaluate the diagnostic precision of the cervical cytology (smear) in a sample of 16 cervical cancer screening centers (CCSCs) from the Mexican Ministry of Health and Mexican Institute for Social Security CCSCs distributed across the country. STUDY DESIGN: Each center received a batch of 90 cytologic specimens with a random positive prevalence of 1.5-36%. Positive cases were always histologically

		confirmed. The "gold standard" was an expert pathologist certified by the Mexican Board of Pathology. RESULTS: Our results show that cytologic diagnosis validity and reproducibility vary greatly within and between institutions. The false negative rate (FNR) varied between 10% and 54%, independent of the prevalence of positive cases. CONCLUSION: Quality control of diagnostic precision is central to the consistency of results obtained at CCSCs. In Mexico the high FNR calls for governmental regulation of cytopathology policies and methods, such as through national and international accreditation of cytotechnology programs. In order to decrease the FNR, developing countries must frame managerial development strategies to streamline the cervical cancer screening program, including continuing education, improvement of operation processes in CCSCs, internal and external quality control of cytopathology laboratories and cervical sampling procedures, and standardization of diagnostic criteria.
	Cytology	Lazcano-Ponce EC Quality control study on negative gynecological cytology in Mexico. Diagn Cytopathol. 1994;10(1):10-4. An external evaluation of the quality of diagnosis of gynecological cytology specimens (Papanicolaou or "Pap" tests) in the Cytopathological Laboratory at the Mexico General Hospital was performed, with evaluation of 6,011 Pap tests randomly selected from 31,378 Pap studies previously reported as negative during 1988-1989. These tests were part of the early detection program for cervical cancer run by the Ministry of Health of Mexico City. A quality index for specimens was constructed based on the presence of endocervical cells, mucus, and squamous metaplastic cells. The index of false negatives for the diagnosis of cervical neoplasm in this sample which correspond to diagnostic error by the examiner was 0.18% (11). The constructed quality index revealed that 64.1% of specimens were low quality. The correlation between diagnostic error and low quality was .87. Results indicate that laboratories participating in early detection programs for cervical cancer in developing countries need to implement (1) external evaluation programs for Pap diagnosis; (2) permanent training programs in registration; and (3) monitoring procedures for collection, fixation, and transportation of cytologic materials.
	Cytology	Lazcano-Ponce E, Alonsa P, Ruiz-Moreno JA, Hernandez-Avila M. Recommendations for cervical cancer screening programs in developing countries. The need for equity and technological development. Salud Publica mex. 2003;45:S3, S449-S62
	HPV	Dzuba IG, Diaz EY et al. The acceptability of self-collected samples for HPV testing vs. the pap test as alternatives in cervical cancer screening. J Womens Health Gend Based Med. 2002 Apr;11(3):265-75 OBJECTIVE: To explore the acceptability of the self-collection of samples for human papillomavirus (HPV) testing in comparison with that of the Pap test. METHODS: The study population consisted of 1069 women 20 years and older who were eligible for coverage through the Mexican Institute of Social Security (IMSS). These women were randomly selected among participants in a larger study to evaluate the use of HPV testing as an alternative in cervical cancer screening. All participants provided a self-collected vaginal sample for HPV testing according to explicit instructions and underwent a Pap test. Afterwards, each woman was interviewed about her experience and opinion regarding the two procedures. Acceptability was

		measured by a calculated score based on discomfort, pain, embarrassment, privacy, perception of personal treatment during the Pap test, and understanding of how to perform the self-sampling method. RESULTS: Ninety-three percent of women experienced sufficient privacy with the Pap test, whereas 98% of women reported that privacy with the self-sampling procedure was acceptable. The Pap test consistently provoked more discomfort, pain, and embarrassment than self-sampling. Sixty-eight percent of the women who indicated a test preference chose self-sampling. Preference for this method was positively associated with monthly household income. Women reported a preference for self-sampling because it is more comfortable (71.2%) and causes less embarrassment (55.8%). CONCLUSIONS: Self-sampling is more acceptable than the Pap test and could improve coverage rates of early detection programs. The incorporation of self-collected samples to detect HPV could encourage participation in screening programs among those women who reject the Pap test because of the necessary pelvic examination.
	Colp	Madrigal de la Campa Mde L, Lazcano-Ponce E, et al Overuse of colposcopy service in Mexico.Ginecol Obstet Mex. 2005 Dec;73(12):637-47 BACKGROUND: Cervicouterine cancer is one of the main public health problems in Mexico. Several problems related to the low effectiveness of the Program of Opportune Detection of Cervicouterine Cancer have been identified, among them: low cover of the disease detection and absence of quality control in the detection, diagnosis and treatment of it. In Mexico the quality control problem in cytology has been taken with success, but the opposite occurs with colposcopy practice. For that reason this service is overused by patients with low risk cancer and is not accessible for the high risk population. OBJECTIVE: To evaluate the association between cervicouterine cancer knowledge and satisfaction with the service regarding the use and intention of adherence to it for the follow-up and treatment, as well as analyze the resources used for this attention. PATIENTS AND METHODS: A transversal study was done from May to December, 2002. It included all the patients who went to the Colposcopy Service in three hospitals. 1,606 patients were interviewed, from them 443 cases were first-time visits and 1,163 were subsequent ones. RESULTS: In a multivariate model we observed that the real utility knowledge of cervicovaginal cytology increases the probability that women come back to the Colposcopy Service (OR 2.0, Cl 95%: 1.57, 2.54). Patients who know their diagnosis when it is dysplasia or cancer are more likely to become attached to their follow-up than those who do not know it. 91% of the users (1,463) had two or more cervicovaginal cytolgies done, and 49% (787) had eight or more. Patients who know the purpose and utility of the biopsy had a 4.4 fold probability of become subsequent than those that do not know such information (Cl 95%: 1.72 to 11.35). CONCLUSIONS: Nowadays colposcopy clinics treat 70% of the patients who are subsequent and that have normal reports of cytology. This shows us an overuse of the service, with the consequent service, monetary and opportunity costs for women. More studies should be done to reformulate the rule that controls the treatment of these patients, and incorporate follow-up guidelines according to the natural history of the disease in Mexican women.
	Pain	http://www.medsch.wisc.edu/painpolicy/publicat/monograp/cmpmexi.htm Graph of Morphine consumption over time

Nicaragua	Stats	Regional Core Health Data Initiative, Pan American Health Organisation, 2003 61.1 new cases per 100,000 population for cervical cancer in Nicaragua 2000
	Recruit	Claeys P, Gonzalez C. et al. Determinants of cervical cancer screening in a resource poor area: results of a population based survey in Rivas, Nicaragua. Tropical Med in International Health. 2002;7(11):935-941 http://www.blackwell-synergy.com/doi/abs/10.1046/j.1365-3156.2002.00953.x?journalCode=tmi&volume=7&issue=11 Inadequate screening is related to low education and lack of knowledge about preventing cancer and its symptoms
	Rural	Howe SL. Cervical cancer prevention in remote rural Nicaragua. Gyn Onc 99(2005)S232-S235 www.icas.net/new-icasweb/docs/Cervical%20cancer%20prevention%20in%20Nicaragua.pdf Nicaragua Ministry of Health, Central American Institute of Health and the Maria Luisa Ortiz clinic undertook a screening project in the rural areas with centralized cytology quality control and co-ordinated treatment. 2132 women were screened with a >95% followthrough rate on treatment of abnormalities.
	Pain	http://www.medsch.wisc.edu/painpolicy/publicat/monograp/cmpnica.htm Graph of Morphine consumption over time
Panama	Stats	Regional Core Health Data Initiative, Pan American Health Organisation, 2003 31.2 new cases per 100,000 population for cervical cancer in Panama 2000
	Pain	http://www.medsch.wisc.edu/painpolicy/publicat/monograp/cmppana.htm Graph of Morphine consumption over time
Paraguay	Stats	Bocciolone L, la Vecchia C, Levi F, Lucchini F, Franceschi S. Trends in uterine cancer mortality in the Americas, 1955–1988. Gynecological Oncology. 1993;51:335–344. http://www.sciencedirect.com/science?_ob=MImg&_imagekey=B6WG6-45PMTSB-9-1&_cdi=6814&_user=10843&_orig=browse&_coverDate=12%2F31%2F1993&_sk=999489996&view=c&wchp=dGLbVtb-zSkzS&md5=db1c792795ed21c919a34a915f9bd853&ie=/sdarticle.pdf Mortality rates were in Paraguay (over 20/100,000). The overall variation in all age-standardized uterine cancer mortality during 1965-1988 (i.e., between 22/100,000 in Paraguay).
	Stats	(Regional Core Health Data Initiative, Pan American Health Organisation, 2003 41.1 new cases per 100,000 population for cervical cancer in Paraguay 2000
	Pain	http://www.medsch.wisc.edu/painpolicy/publicat/monograp/cmppara.htm Graph of Morphine consumption over time
Peru	Stats	Regional Core Health Data Initiative, Pan American Health Organisation, 2003 39.9 new cases per 100,000 population for cervical cancer in Peru 2000
	Stats	*Source:* Parkin et al. (eds.) Cancer Incidence in Five Continents (Vol. V, VI, VII) Malignant Neoplasm of the *Cervix uteri:*Average Annual Age-Standardized Incidence Rates
	Recrut	Hunter J. Cervical cancer in Iquito Peru local realities to guide prevention

		planning. Cad Salud Publica 2004;20(1):160-171 Misconception that pap identifies cancer rather than preventing it.
	Recruit	Aguito I, Bishop A. Perceived barriers and benefits of cervical cancer screening in Latin America. Preventive Medicine 2004;49:91-8 http://www.sciencedirect.com/science?_ob=MImg&_imagekey=B6WPG-4CCF94C-2-1&_cdi=6990&_user=10843&_orig=browse&_coverDate=07%2F31%2F2004&_sk=999609998&view=c&wchp=dGLbVzz-zSkWW&md5=ff06818626496f2eeeebbd037e0db590&ie=/sdarticle.pdf Except for the accessibility and availability of quality services, these results are consistent with findings from other studies in developed and developing countries. Barriers could be lifted if health service delivery was enhanced, for instance, through quality improvement techniques that are available at low cost. Women's anxiety over test results still needs to be further assessed to devise risk communication strategies that take into account broader cultural frameworks. It is to be noted that such strategies should permeate the way health services are provided for cervical cancer prevention regardless of the specific test used. Vulnerability perceived by low-income women with respect to their capacity to cope with diseases and trust the health services and how this affects their perceptions of risk and their behaviors have not been studied as yet.
	Screening VIA+PAP	http://www.paho.org/English/DD/PIN/01_ARTI_Jeronimo--1-5.pdf pdf of article by Jeronima J. from NIH USA on VIA for cervix cancer screening outside low resource settings. Pan Am J Public Health 17(1)2005 VIA is useful for detection of precursor lesions of cervical cancer not only in low resource setting but in well equipped health centres and cancer centres. In these non-low resource settings, VIA has a PPV comparable to conventional PAP but it is more likely to achieve earlier diagnosis, follow-up and treatment than cytology based screening.
	Treatment	http://www.path.org/files/RH_supporting_women_iid.pdf Problems with transportation of patients to urban areas for treatment
	Radiation therapy	CRP Number and Title: E33012 Clinical application of radiosensitizers in cancer radiotherapy Participating Countries: Austria(C), Austria(C), China(C), India(C), Japan(A), Japan(A), Japan(C), Nigeria(C), Pakistan(C), Peru(C), Sri Lanka(C), Turkey(C), United Kingdom(C) Total Cost: $273 614 Duration: 1994-09-15 – 2002-12-31 CRP Overall Objectives To study the Clinical Application of Radiosensitizers in Cancer Radiotherapy. CRP Specific Objectives To conduct an international multicentre randomized clinical trial. of a hypoxic cell radiosensitiser, AK-2123 in the treatment of cervix cancer. Research Outputs From 19 May 1995 to 16 December 1998, 333 patients were randomised and treated either by radical radiotherapy (RT) or radiotherapy with the addition of a hypoxic cell radiosensitiser, AK-2123. Six patients were excluded as they were never treated and were lost to follow up. Local toxicity did not differ significantly in the two treatment groups.

		There were 20 patients in the RT+AK-2123 arm who experienced peripheral neuropathy. In most cases, this normalized within 6 months. In one patient a mild, permanent peripheral neuropathy has been recorded. The rate of local tumour control was 62% after RT+AK-2123 and 46% after RT (p=0.006), which is significant. The actuarial survival at 60 months was 57% after RT+AK-2123, compared to 41% after RT (Log Rank p= 0.007). CRP Outcome (Effectiveness; Impact; Relevance) The CRP has been concluded and the preliminary results are encouraging. This clinical trial has advanced the study of Clinical Application of Radiosensitizers in Cancer Radiotherapy The low toxicity and improved tumor control are encouraging but the short follow-up of the patients would need to extended for critical acceptance. Recommended Future Action by Agency 1. The Agency needs to provide for sophisticated support by statisticians in such studies. 2. After the independent expert peer-reviewers' comments/criticisms are received from the International Journal of Radiation Oncology Biology and Physics, additional funding may be necessary to address those comments/criticisms. CRP Published Results The manuscript was submitted in Oct 2002 to the International Journal of Radiation Oncology Biology and Physics.
	Pain	http://www.medsch.wisc.edu/painpolicy/publicat/monograp/cmpperu.htm Graph of Morphine consumption over time
Puerto Rico	Stats	*Source:* Parkin et al. (eds.) Cancer Incidence in Five Continents (Vol. V, VI, VII Malignant Neoplasm of the *Cervix uteri:* Average Annual Age-Standardized Incidence Rates (per 100,000 inhabitants, selected countries of the Americas, 1978-1992)
	Stats	Regional Core Health Data Initiative, Pan American Health Organisation, 2003 10.3 new cases per 100,000 population for cervical cancer in Puerto Rico 2000
	Stats	Bocciolone L, la Vecchia C, Levi F, Lucchini F, Franceschi S. Trends in uterine cancer mortality in the Americas, 1955–1988. Gynecological Oncology. 1993;51:335–344. doi: 10.1006/gyno.1993.1300. http://www.sciencedirect.com/science?_ob=MImg&_imagekey=B6WG6-45PMTSB-9-1&_cdi=6814&_user=10843&_orig=browse&_coverDate=12%2F31%2F1993&_sk=999489996&view=c&wchp=dGLbVtb-zSkzS&md5=db1c792795ed21c919a34a915f9bd853&ie=/sdarticle.pdf
Surinam	Stats	Regional Core Health Data Initiative, Pan American Health Organization, 2003 43.8 new cases per 100,000 population for cervical cancer in Suriname 2000
	Stats	High cervical cancer rates Incidence: 43/100,000
	HPV type	Krul EJ, Van De Vijver MH, Schuuring E. Human papillomavirus in malignant cervical lesions in Surinam, a high-risk country, compared to the Netherlands, a low-risk country. Int J Gynecol Cancer. 1999 May;9(3):206-211.

		http://www.blackwell-synergy.com/doi/abs/10.1046/j.1525-1438.1999.99020.x?journalCode=ijg&volume=9&issue=3 We determined the presence of HPV and the distribution of the different HPV genotypes in cervical carcinomas from Surinam, a high-incidence country. The results were compared to the Netherlands where the incidence is five times lower. One hundred thirty cervical carcinomas from patients in Surinam were randomly selected and compared to an unselected group of 128 cervical carcinomas from caucasoid Dutch patients. Presence of HPV and distribution of HPV genotypes was determined in DNA extracted from paraffin-embedded specimens by polymerase chain reaction and sequence analysis. HPV DNA was detected in 82% of the Surinamese cervical cancer patients and in 87% of the Dutch patients. Thirteen different HPV genotypes were detected in the Surinamese group, and nine different HPV genotypes were detected in the Dutch group. Among the HPV-positive samples, HPV 16 was present in 68% in the Netherlands compared to only 49% in Surinam, where less common genotypes such as HPV 35, 45, and 58 were more prevalent. The results show a strong association between HPV and cervical cancer in both groups. However, the observed significant variation in distribution of the genotypes in the two populations with a large difference in cervical carcinoma incidence is important to the general understanding of the etiology of cervical cancer and to the development of HPV vaccination strategies.
Trinidad and Tobago	Stats	Regional Core Health Data Initiative, Pan American Health Organisation, 2003 33.3 new cases per 100,000 population for cervical cancer in Trinidad and Tobago 2000
Uruguary	Stats	Bocciolone L, la Vecchia C, Levi F, Lucchini F, Franceschi S. Trends in uterine cancer mortality in the Americas, 1955–1988. Gynecological Oncology. 1993;51:335–344. http://www.sciencedirect.com/science?_ob=MImg&_imagekey=B6WG6-45PMTSB-9-1&_cdi=6814&_user=10843&_orig=browse&_coverDate=12%2F31%2F1993&_sk=999489996&view=c&wchp=dGLbVtb-zSkzS&md5=db1c792795ed21c919a34a915f9bd853&ie=/sdarticle.pdf Over the last two decades most Latin American countries showed declines in mortality rates ranging of 25-35% in Uruguay.
	Stats	Regional Core Health Data Initiative, Pan American Health Organisation, 2003 13.8 new cases per 100,000 population for cervical cancer in Uruguay 2000
Venezeula	Stats	Regional Core Health Data Initiative, Pan American Health Organisation, 2003 38.3 new cases per 100,000 population for cervical cancer in Venezuela 2000
	Screening	Aguito I, Bishop A. Perceived barriers and benefits of cervical cancer screening in Latin America. Preventive Medicine 2004;49:91-8 http://www.sciencedirect.com/science?_ob=MImg&_imagekey=B6WPG-4CCF94C-2-1&_cdi=6990&_user=10843&_orig=browse&_coverDate=07%2F31%2F2004&_sk=999609998&view=c&wchp=dGLbVzz-zSkWW&md5=ff06818626496f2eeeebbd037e0db590&ie=/sdarticle.pdf

		Except for the accessibility and availability of quality services, these results are consistent with findings from other studies in developed and developing countries. Barriers could be lifted if health service delivery was enhanced, for instance, through quality improvement techniques that are available at low cost. Women's anxiety over test results still needs to be further assessed to devise risk communication strategies that take into account broader cultural frameworks. It is to be noted that such strategies should permeate the way health services are provided for cervical cancer prevention regardless of the specific test used. Vulnerability perceived by low-income women with respect to their capacity to cope with diseases and trust the health services and how this affects their perceptions of risk and their behaviors have not been studied as yet.
	Screening	http://ncd.bvsalud.org/portals/cervicalCancer/docs/en/VenezuelaCC.doc (Spanish)
	Pain	http://www.medsch.wisc.edu/painpolicy/publicat/monograp/cmpvene.htm Graph of Morphine consumption over time
	Pain	http://www.medsch.wisc.edu/painpolicy/publicat/monograp/encvene.htm Graph of Morphine needs versus consumption
	Stats	Bocciolone L, la Vecchia C, Levi F, Lucchini F, Franceschi S. Trends in uterine cancer mortality in the Americas, 1955–1988. Gynecological Oncology. 1993;51:335–344. doi: 10.1006/gyno.1993.1300. (Pdf of article) http://www.sciencedirect.com/science?_ob=MImg&_imagekey=B6WG6-45PMTSB-9-1&_cdi=6814&_user=10843&_orig=browse&_coverDate=12%2F31%2F1993&_sk=999489996&view=c&wchp=dGLbVtb-zSkzS&md5=db1c792795ed21c919a34a915f9bd853&ie=/sdarticle.pdf Over the last two decades most Latin American countries showed declines in mortality rates ranging of 25-35% in Venuzuela.

SECTION 3 : EDUCATIONAL MATERIAL RELATED TO CERVICAL CANCER

To be included in this compendium the material was 1) developed by an international agency, or 2) if developed by a high resource setting there was evidence that it was assessed in a low resource setting or 3) available in languages other than English, and developed since the year 2000. The materials listed here are available in a variety of formats such as manuals, fast fact sheets, presentations, training manuals. Where materials are available in multiple languages we have indicated this.

Agency – indicates the host publisher.

Audience-the most likely group to benefit from being aware of this information

(c) – year the material was copyrighted

List of Organizations which have published on cervix cancer control

International Organization	Link
ACCP	http://www.alliance-cxca.org/english/publications.html#cciid
EngenderHealth	http://search.atomz.com/search/?sp-q=cervix+cancer&sp-a=sp1000b9b8
JHPIEGO	http://www.jhpiego.org/scripts/pubs/product_search.asp
IAEA	http://www.iaea.org/Publications/Training/index.html
IARC	http://www.iarc.fr/cgi-bin/htsearch
ISNCC	http://www.isncc.org/lists.asp?table=Publications
PAHO	http://www.paho.org/Selection.asp?SEL=PR&LNG=ENG
PATH	http://search.atomz.com/search/?sp-a=00040367-sp00000001&sp-q=cervix+cancer
WHO	http://search.who.int/search?ie=utf8&site=default_collection&client=WHO&proxystylesheet=WHO&output=xml_no_dtd&oe=utf8&q=cervix+cancer http://www.who.int/bookorders/anglais/catalog_suj1.jsp?sesslan=1&hidsubject=70100

Areas

1. Educational Tools on Cancer Control Programs for Low Resource Settings

Agency	Audience	Item
WHO	Policy Makers	Cancer Control: Knowledge into action. WHO guide for effective programmes ©2006 http://www.who.int/bookorders/anglais/detart1.jsp?sesslan=1&codlan=1&codcol=15&codcch=674
NIH	Policy Makers	Disease Control Priorities in Developing Countries Chap 29: health Service Intervention for Cancer Control in developing Countries © 2006 http://www.ncbi.nlm.nih.gov/books/bv.fcgi?rid=dcp2.chapter.4129
WHO	Policy Makers	National Cancer Control Program: Policies and Managerial Guidelines. 2nd ed © 2002 http://www.who.int/cancer/media/en/408.pdf

2. Educational Tools on Cervical Cancer Control Programs for Low Resource Settings

Agency	Audience	Web Line
WHO	Policy Makers Health Care Providers Managers	Comprehensive Cervical Cancer Control © 2006 http://www.who.int/reproductive-health/publications/cervical_cancer_gep/index.htm
IARC	Health Care Providers	Cervix cancer screening © 2005 http://www.iarc.fr/IARCPress/pdfs/handbook10/HANDBOOK10.pdf (17MB)
ACCP		Planning and Implementing cervical cancer prevention and control programs: A manual for managers © 2004 http://www.who.int/reproductive-health/cancers/prevention_control_cervical_cancer.html (3.89MB)

		English, Spanish, French, Russian
ACCP	Policy Makers	Preventing Cervical Cancer Worldwide © 2004 http://www.path.org/files/RH_prp-accp_cervical_cancer_worldw.pdf English http://www.prb.org/pdf05/PreventCervCancer_SP.pdf Spanish http://www.prb.org/pdf05/PreventCervCancer_FR.pdf French
ACCP	Policy Makers	Cervical Cancer Fact Sheet © 2004 http://www.path.org/files/RH_conclusions.pdf English http://www.path.org/files/RH_accp_conclusions_fs_fr.pdf French http://www.path.org/files/RH_accp_conclusions_fs_sp.pdf Spanish
ACCP	Policy Makers	A Case for investing in Cervix Cancer © 2004 http://www.path.org/files/RH_accp_case.pdf
WHO	Policy Makers	Cervical Cancer Screening in Developing Countries © 2002 http://www.who.int/cancer/media/en/cancer_cervical_37321.pdf
EngenderHealth	Manager	COPE ® for Cervical Cancer Prevention Services: A Toolbook to Accompany the COPE® Handbook. © 2004 A supplement to COPE® Handbook: A Process for Improving Quality in Health Services, Revised Edition. Provides updated versions of the self-assessment guides, the client interview guide, and other materials for identifying and solving on-site problems that compromise the quality of cervical cancer prevention services. Among the cervical cancer-specific issues addressed in the tools are screening tests and examinations, laboratory services, treatment of precancerous lesions, appropriate follow-up and management of clients, referral and feedback between different service components, and equipment and supplies http://www.engenderhealth.org/res/offc/qi/cope/toolbook/pdf/cope_cxca_toolbook.pdf Pilot tested in Bolivia English, Spanish
PATH	Policy Makers	Planning Appropriate Cervical Cancer Prevention Programs © 2000 http://www.path.org/files/cxca-planning-appro-prog-guide.pdf
RHO	Power point presentation	Planning Appropriate Cervical Cancer Control Programs © 1998 http://www.rho.org/html/cxca_planningdocument.htm

3. Educational Tools on Epidemiology

Agency	**Audience**	**Resource**
ASCCP	Patient	What women should know about HPV and cervical health http://www.asccp.org/pdfs/patient_edu/women_should_know.pdf *English* 5 page pamphlet http://www.asccp.org/pdfs/patient_edu/spanish/HPV.pdf *Spanish* 4 page pamphlet
CDC	Patient	HPV: Common Infection, common reality http://www.cdc.gov/std/hpv/common-infection/HPVBrochureCleared-Online.pdf 8 page pamphlet
ACCP	Health Care Providers	Risk Factors for Cervical cancer: Evidence to date © 2004 http://www.path.org/files/RH_fs_risk_factors.pdf *English* http://www.path.org/files/RH_risk_factors_fs_sp.pdf *Spanish* http://www.path.org/files/RH_risk_factors_fs_fr.pdf *French*

JHPEIGO	Patients and Health Care Providers	HPV and Cervix Cancer information sheet http://www.reproline.jhu.edu/english/3cc/3refman/cxca_hpv1.htm
CDC	Patient	Genital HPV Infection http://www.cdc.gov/std/HPV/STDFact-HPV.htm *English* http://www.cdc.gov/std/Spanish/STDFact-HPV-s.htm *Spanish*
NCI	Patients	Human Papillomavirus and Cancer: Questions and Answers http://www.cancer.gov/cancertopics/factsheet/Risk/HPV
NCCC	Patients	Human Papillomavirus and Genital Warts © 2006 http://www.niaid.nih.gov/factsheets/stdhpv.htm English, Spanish
OncoLink	Patients	HPV and Cervix Cancer © 2005 http://www.oncolink.com/types/article.cfm?c=6&s=17&ss=131&id=9 531

4. Educational Material on Primary Prevention

Agency	**Audience**	**Web link**
WHO	Policy makers	Preparing for the introduction of HPV vaccines: policy and programme guidance for countries © 2006 http://www.who.int//reproductive-health/publications/hpvvaccines/index.html
PATH	Decision Makers	Cervical cancer vaccine project http://www.path.org/files/RH_cc_vacc_proj_fs.pdf
PATH	Decision makers	Status report on vaccines http://www.path.org/files/RH_HPV_status_report.pdf
IARC	Decision makers	Kols A, Sherris J. HPV Vaccines: Promises and Challenges © 2000 http://screening.iarc.fr/doc/jsrp13710.pdf
CDC	Health Care Providers	HPV and HPV Vaccine http://www.cdc.gov/std/hpv/STDFact-HPV-vaccine-hcp.htm
SGO	Patients	You can prevent cervix cancer http://www.cervicalcancercampaign.org/vaccine_FAQ.aspx
SGO	Patient	You can prevent cervix cancer http://www.wcn.org/CC_Vaccine_Brochure.pdf
ASHA	Patients	FAQs about Cervical Cancer/HPV vaccine access in the USA http://www.ashastd.org/pdfs/FAQ_HPV_0606.pdf

5. Information Systems

Agency	**Audience**	**Web link**
PAHO	IT	Improving country programs via a cervical cancer information system: a tool for program management and evaluation http://www.paho.org/English/AD/DPC/NC/ccimprovingcountryprog.doc

IT-Information Technology

6. Screening

Agency	**Audience**	**Web link**
Eurogin	Health care providers	HPV DNA testing in cervical cancer screening: From evidence to policies © 2006

		http://www.sciencedirect.com/science?_ob=MImg&_imagekey=B6WG6-4KPFKDD-4-1&_cdi=6814&_user=10843&_orig=browse&_coverDate=10%2F31%2F2006&_sk=998969998&view=c&wchp=dGLbVlz-zSkzk&md5=cfdac69d441da9e9394586a3ecbb4496&ie=/sdarticle.pdf
WHO	Health Care Providers	Cervix cancer Screening: IARC Handbook on Cancer Prevention #19 © 2005 http://www.who.int/bookorders/anglais/detart1.jsp?sesslan=1&codlan=1&codcol=76&codcch=18
ACCP	Managers	Planning and Implementing cervical cancer prevention and control programs © 2004 http://www.afro.who.int/cdp/documents/cervical_cancer/ACCP%20manuel_1.pdf
ACCP	Health care providers	Cervical Cancer Prevention Fact Sheet © 2004 http://www.path.org/files/RH_conclusions.pdf
ACCP	Pdf or power point	Developing cervix cancer Screening Programs that meet women's needs © 2003 http://www.path.org/files/RH_meeting_womens_needs.pdf *English* http://www.path.org/files/RH_meeting_womens_needs_fr.pdf *French* http://www.path.org/files/RH_meeting_womens_needs_sp.pdf *Spanish*
IARC	Powerpoint	Screening options http://www.alliance-cxca.org/files/Sankar_FIGO.pdf
NCI	Patients	Understanding Cervical Changes: A health guide for women
ACCP	Health Care Providers	Sankaranarayanan R, Gaffiken L, Jacob M, Sellors J, Robles S. A critical assessment of screening methods for cervical neoplasia. Int J Gyn Ob 2005;89:S4-S12 http://www.womenshealth-elsevier.com/doc/journals/ijgo_si_89-2/02.pdf
ACCP	Health Care Providers	Bradley J, Barone M, Mahe C, Lewis R, Luciani S. Delivering cervical cancer prevention services in low resource settings. Int J Gyn Ob 2005;89:S21-S29
ACCP	Public Policy Makers	Sherris J, Agurto I, Arrossi S, Dzuba I, Gaffiken L, Herdman C, Limpaphayom K, Luciani S. Advocating for cervical cancer prevention. Int J Gyn Ob 2005;89:S46-S54 http://www.womenshealth-elsevier.com/doc/journals/ijgo_si_89-2/06.pdf
ACCP	Public Policy Makers	Tsu VD, Pollock AE. Preventing Cervical cancer in Low resource settings: How far have we come and what does the future hold. Int J Gyn Ob 2005;89:S55-S59 http://www.womenshealth-elsevier.com/doc/journals/ijgo_si_89-2/09.pdf
ACCP	Public Policy Makers	Program capacity assessment tool: Integrating cervical cancer prevention into reproductive health services © 2001 http://www.path.org/files/Tool-16-july.pdf
JHPIEGO	Health Care Providers	This handbook for participants describes a competency-based training course and includes the course objectives, model course schedule, learning guides and practice checklists, and instructions for using the ZOE® anatomic model, all linked to

		the reference manual. © 2005 http://www.jhpiego.org/scripts/pubs/product_detail.asp?product_id=553
JHPIEGO	Trainers and Health Care Providers	This reference manual is designed for trainers and health care providers who are embarking on a cervical cancer prevention program that will focus on visual inspection with acetic acid (VIA) and/or cryotherapy as the core programmatic elements. The material is arranged both according to established principles of medical education (epidemiology, pathophysiology, clinical intervention) and according to the order in which knowledge and skills are gradually acquired during training. Although this manual could be used alone in training in provision of VIA and cryotherapy services, it is an integral part of a comprehensive learning package that includes a handbook for participants, a notebook for trainers, an interactive CD-ROM of cervical images, a companion handbook on performance support and anatomic models © 2005 http://www.jhpiego.org/scripts/pubs/product_detail.asp?product_id=532
JHPIEGO	Trainers and Health Care Providers	This notebook for trainers contains the precourse and midcourse questionnaires and answer keys, detailed course outline and competency-based qualifications checklists, in addition to all participant material. Handbooks and notebooks are usually provide © 2005 http://www.jhpiego.org/scripts/pubs/product_detail.asp?product_id=554
AICR	Patients	Cervix Cancer http://www.aicr.org.uk/CervicalCancerFA.stm
JHPIEGO	Quality assurance	The purpose of this handbook, developed for use in conjunction with the training manual Cervical Cancer Prevention Guidelines for Low-Resource Settings, is to provide guidance to anyone who is responsible for performance support and/or quality assurance for cervical prevention services based on visual inspection using acetic acid (VIA) and cryotherapy. © 2005 http://www.jhpiego.org/scripts/pubs/product_detail.asp?product_id=555

7. Community, Educate the Public

Agency	**Audience**	**Reference**
ACCP	Managers	Agurto I, Arrossi S, White S, Coffey P, Dzuba I, Bingham A, Bradley J, Lewis R. Involving the community in cervical cancer prevention programs. Int J Gyn Ob 2005;89:S38-S45 http://www.womenshealth-elsevier.com/doc/journals/ijgo_si_89-2/06.pdf
ACCP	Managers	Key steps – Fast Fact Sheet © 2002 http://www.path.org/files/RH_key_steps_fs.pdf *English* http://www.path.org/files/RH_key_steps_fs_fr.pdf *French* http://www.path.org/files/RH_key_steps_sp_fs.pdf *Spanish* http://www.path.org/files/RH_key_steps_fs_r.pdf *Russian*
ACCP	Health Care Providers	Questions women frequently ask © 2003 http://www.path.org/files/RH_faq_fs.pdf *English*

		http://www.path.org/files/RH_questions_asked_fs_fr.pdf *French* http://www.path.org/files/RH_questions_asked_fs_sp.pdf *Spanish* http://www.path.org/files/RH_questions_asked_fs_fr.pdf *Russian*
ACCP	Pdf and Power point	Women's Frequently Asked Questions About Cervical Cancer Screening: Helping Health Care Providers Anticipate and Answer Common Questions. © 2003 http://www.path.org/files/RH_womens_faqs.pdf *English* http://www.path.org/files/RH_womens_faqs_sp.pdf *Spanish* http://www.path.org/files/RH_womens_faqs_fr.pdf *French*
ACCP	Public Policy	Improving Screening Coverage Rates of Cervix Cancer Prevention Programs © 2004 http://www.path.org/files/RH_accp_improve_screening.pdf
ACCP	Community education	Republic of Peru: National Program for Gynecologic Cancer Prevention. A guide for community facilitation. http://www.path.org/files/RH_prevent_cc.pdf

8. Pelvic Examination and Pap Test

Agency	**Audience**	**Resource**
PAHO	Patient	Counseling tool for patients – developed in El Salvador http://www.paho.org/English/AD/DPC/NC/pcc-afiche.htm
ASCCP	Patient	Smoking and Pap test http://www.asccp.org/pdfs/patient_edu/Smoking_and_Pap.pdf *English*
ACCP	Health Care Provider and Patient	Natural History of Cervical Cancer Screening http://www.path.org/files/RH_natural_history_of_cc_fs.pdf *English* http://www.path.org/files/cxca-factsheet-natural-history-SPAN.pdf *Spanish* http://www.path.org/files/RH_natural_history_fs_fr.pdf *French* http://www.path.org/files/RH_natural_history_fs_r.pdf *Russian*
ACCP	Health Care Providers	Pap smear: Important but imperfect method © 2002, http://www.path.org/files/RH_pap_smears.pdf *English* http://www.path.org/files/RH_pap_smears_sp.pdf *Spanish* http://www.path.org/files/RH_pap_smears_fs_fr.pdf *French* http://www.path.org/files/RH_pap_smears_fs_r.pdf *Russian*
ACCP	Pdf or Powerpoint	The Pap Test: Evidence to date http://www.path.org/files/RH_pap_test.pdf *English* http://www.path.org/files/RH_pap_presentation_sp.pdf *Spanish* http://www.path.org/files/RH_pap_test_fr.pdf *French*
ACS	Patient	What is a Pap test? http://www.cancer.org/docroot/PED/content/PED_2_3X_Pap_Test.asp?sitearea=PED
ACS	Patient	Cancer Facts for Women http://www.cancer.org/downloads/asn/CanFactsWom_Eng.pdf English http://www.cancer.org/downloads/ASN/CanFactsWom_Chin.pdf Chinese http://www.cancer.org/downloads/ASN/CanFactsWom_Kor.pdf Korean http://www.cancer.org/downloads/asn/CanFactsWom_Viet.pdf Vietnamese
CDC	Patient	Basic Facts on screening and the Pap smear

		http://www.cdc.gov/cancer/nbccedp/bccpdfs/cc_basic.pdf
NCI	Patient	Pap smear http://www.cancer.gov/cancertopics/factsheet/Detection/Pap-test
NCI	Patient	Understand cervix changes: a Health guide for women 23 pages http://www.cancer.gov/cancertopics/understandingcervicalchangesPDF
OncoLink	Patient	Pap Test: Cervical Changes © 2002 http://www.oncolink.com/types/article.cfm?c=6&s=17&ss=131&id=60 27
NCCC	Patient	http://www.iwannaknow.org/basics2/hpv.html

9. Cytology

Agency	Audience	Resource
IARC	Pathology Cytology	Frappart L, Frontaniere B, Lucas E, Sankaranyanan R. Histopathology and cytopathology of the uterine cervix. Digital atlas 2004. http://screening.iarc.fr/atlashisto.php?lang=1&PHPSESSID=75e4f30359 dc9b176ebd12a697bc4ad7
USCAP	Cytology	Short courses in gynecologic pathology listed under educational materials http://www.uscap.org/
IAC	Cytology	NCI Bethesda System http://www.cytopathology.org/NIH/index.php
CAP	Cytology	Resource list http://www.cap.org/apps/cap.portal?_nfpb=true&cntvwrPtlt_actionOver ride=%2Fportlets%2FcontentViewer%2Fshow&_windowLabel=cntvwr Ptlt&cntvwrPtlt%7BactionForm.contentReference%7D=disciplines%2F cytopathology%2Fcytopathology_index.html&_state=maximized&_pag eLabel=cntvwr

10. HPV Testing

Agency	Audience	Resource
EUROGIN	Health Care Providers	HPV DNA testing in cervical cancer screening: From evidence to policies http://www.sciencedirect.com/science?_ob=MImg&_imagekey=B6 WG6-4KPFKDD-4-1&_cdi=6814&_user=10843&_orig=browse&_coverDate=10%2F31 %2F2006&_sk=998969998&view=c&wchp=dGLbVlz-zSkzk&md5=cfdac69d441da9e9394586a3ecbb4496&ie=/sdarticle.pd f
ASCCP	Patient	HPV testing http://www.asccp.org/pdfs/patient_edu/hpv_testing.pdf
ACCP	Health Care Provider	HPV testing – Fact sheet ©2003 http://www.path.org/files/RH_hpv_testing_fs.pdf *English* http://www.path.org/files/RH_hpv_testing_fs_sp.pdf *Spanish* http://www.path.org/files/RH_hpv_testing_fs_fr.pdf *French* http://www.path.org/files/RH_hpv_testing_fs_r.pdf *Russian*

11. Educational Material on VIA

Agency	Audience	Resource
PAHO	Health Care providers	Visual Inspection of the uterine cervix with acetic acid (VIA): A critical review of selected articles © 2003 http://www.paho.org/English/AD/DPC/NC/cc-via.pdf
ACCP	Health Care Providers	Blumenthal P, Lauterbach M, Sellors JW, Sankaranarayanan R. Training for cervical cancer prevention programs in low resource settings: focus on visual inspection with acetic acid and cryotherapy. Int J Gyn Ob 2005;89:S30-S37 http://www.womenshealth-elsevier.com/doc/journals/ijgo_si_89-2/05.pdf
ACCP	Health Care Providers	VIA – an alternate approach © 2002 http://www.path.org/files/RH_visual_screening.pdf *English* http://www.path.org/files/RH_visual_sp_fs.pdf *Spanish* http://www.path.org/files/RH_visual_screening_fs_fr.pdf *French* http://www.path.org/files/RH_visual_screening_fs_r.pdf *Russian*
ACCP	Pdf or powerpoint	Visual inspection with acetic acid (VIA): Evidence to date http://www.path.org/files/RH_via_evidence.pdf *English* http://www.path.org/files/RH_via_presentation_sp.pdf *Spanish* http://www.path.org/files/RH_via_evidence_fr.pdf *French*
ACCP	Pdf or powerpoint	Visual inspection with Lugol's iodine (VILI): Evidence to date http://www.path.org/files/RH_vili.pdf *English* http://www.path.org/files/RH_vili_presentation_sp.pdf *Spanish* http://www.path.org/files/RH_vili_fr.pdf *French*
IARC	Health Care Provider	Sankaranarayanan R, Wesley S. A Practical Manual on Visual Screening for cervix neoplasia. © 2003 http://screening.iarc.fr/viavili.php?lang=1&PHPSESSID=75e4f3035 9dc9b176ebd12a697bc4ad7

12. Other Technologies

Agency	Item	Resource
PATH	Fast Fact Sheet	Innovation in other technologies © 2006 http://www.path.org/files/RH_start_biochem_scr_fs_en.pdf
ACCP	Pdf or powerpoint	Researching new prevention approaches for cervical cancer: Methodological guidelines http://www.path.org/files/RH_research_methods.pdf *English* http://www.path.org/files/RH_research_methods_sp.pdf *Spanish* http://www.path.org/files/RH_research_methods_fr.ppt*French*
PATH	Fast Fact Sheet	Rapid HPV Test © 2006 http://www.path.org/files/TS_update_cervical_cancer.pdf Chinese, English

13. Colposcopy

Agency	Audience	Resource
ASCCP	Patient	Colposcopy http://www.asccp.org/pdfs/patient_edu/spanish/colposcopy.pdf

		English, Spanish
ASCCP	Colposcopists	HPV training course http://cme.asccp.org/home/home.cfm
IARC	Physicians	Colposcopy and Treatment of Cervical Intraepithelial Neoplasia: A Beginner's Manual Sellors JW, Sankaranarayanan R. Lyon, France: IARC (2003). Non-Serial Publication ISBN 92 832 0412, I.A.R.C. Press. www.iarc.fr/pageroot/PUBLICATIONS/howtoorder.pdf
Oncolink	Patient	Colposcopy http://www.oncolink.com/types/article.cfm?c=6&s=17&ss=131&id=6028
IFCPC ASCCP	Physicians	On line CME courses 1credit per coarse http://cme.asccp.org/cme/CMECourseList.cfm
IFCPC	Physicians	Compendium of Colposcopy images from France http://www.ifcpc.org/ifcpc/education_colpophoto.htm *French*

14. Treatment for Abnormal Pap

Agency	**Audience**	**Procedure**	**Resource**
ASCCP	Patients	Cone	http://www.asccp.org/pdfs/patient_edu/cone_biopsy.pdf *English* http://www.asccp.org/pdfs/patient_edu/spanish/cone_biopsy.pdf *Spanish*
ASCCP	Patients	LEEP	http://www.asccp.org/pdfs/patient_edu/leep.pdf *English* http://www.asccp.org/pdfs/patient_edu/spanish/LEEP.pdf *Spanish*
ASCCP	Patients	Cryotherapy	http://www.asccp.org/pdfs/patient_edu/spanish/cervical_cryotherapy.pdf *English* http://www.asccp.org/pdfs/patient_edu/spanish/cervical_cryotherapy.pdf *Spanish*
ACCP	Health care Providers	Cryotherapy	Jacob M, Broekheizen FF, Castro W, Sellors J. Experience using cryotherapy for treatment of cervical precancer lesions in low resource settings. Int J Gyn Ob 2005;89:S113-S20. http://www.womenshealth-elsevier.com/doc/journals/ijgo_si_89-2/03.pdf
ACCP	Health Care Providers	Cryo and LEEP	Treatment options http://www.path.org/files/RH_treatment_fs.pdf *English* http://www.path.org/files/RH_lesions_fs_sp.pdf *Spanish* http://www.path.org/files/RH_cervical_lesions_fs_fr.pdf *French* http://www.path.org/files/RH_treatment_fs_r.pdf *Russian*
ACCP	Powerpt	Cryotherapy	http://www.alliance-cxca.org/files/PB_FIGO_Cryo_ACCP.pdf
OncoLink	Patient	LEEP	http://www.oncolink.com/types/article.cfm?c=6&s=17&ss=131&id=6026

15. Cancer

Agency	**Audience**	**Resource**
Gynecologic Cancer Foundation	Public	Understanding Cervical Cancer
ACS	Public	All About Cervix Cancer website http://www.cancer.org/docroot/CRI/CRI_2x.asp?sitearea=&dt=8
ACS	Public	Overview http://www.cancer.org/downloads/PRO/CervicalCancer.pdf
CCS	Public	What is Cervical Cancer? http://www.cancer.ca/ccs/survey/P5Frames.asp?source=http%3A%2F%2Fwww%2Ecancer%2Eca%2Fccs%2Finternet%2Ffrontdoor%2F0%2C%2C3543%5F%5F%5FlangId%2Den%2C00%2Ehtml&site=1&lang=EN&log=235083 English, French
CCS	Public	Cervix Cancer: What you need to know? http://www.cancer.ca/vgn/images/portal/cit_86751114/63/40/151140772cw_library_wyntk_cervical_en.pdf *English* http://www.cancer.ca/vgn/images/portal/cit_86755361/9/14/155834523cw_library_Cervicalwyntk_fr.pdf *French* http://www.cancer.ca/ccs/survey/P5Frames.asp?source=http%3A%2F%2Fwww%2Ecancer%2Eca%2Fccs%2Finternet%2Ffrontdoor%2F0%2C%2C3543%5F%5F%5FlangId%2Den%2C00%2Ehtml&site=1&lang=EN&log=235083 *Chinese* http://www.cancer.ca/ccs/survey/P5Frames.asp?source=http%3A%2F%2Fwww%2Ecancer%2Eca%2Fccs%2Finternet%2Ffrontdoor%2F0%2C%2C3543%5F%5F%5FlangId%2Den%2C00%2Ehtml&site=1&lang=EN&log=235083 *Farsi* http://www.cancer.ca/ccs/survey/P5Frames.asp?source=http%3A%2F%2Fwww%2Ecancer%2Eca%2Fccs%2Finternet%2Ffrontdoor%2F0%2C%2C3543%5F%5F%5FlangId%2Den%2C00%2Ehtml&site=1&lang=EN&log=235083 *Punjabi*
NCI	Health Care Provider	Cervix Cancer http://www.cancer.gov/cancertopics/types/cervical/
ACOG	Patient	Cervix Cancer http://www.acog.org/publications/patient_education/bp163.cfm
Oncolink	Patient	Cervix Cancer http://www.oncolink.com/types/article.cfm?c=6&s=17&ss=129&id=8226
College of American Pathologists	Pathology	Check list only http://www.cap.org/apps/docs/cancer_protocols/2005/uterinecervix05_ckw.pdf Full protocol:Uterine cervix http://www.cap.org/apps/docs/cancer_protocols/2005/uterinecervix05_pw.pdf

16. Radiation Treatment

Focus	Audience	Resource and Link
Brachytherapy	Radiation Oncologists and Technologists	The GEC ESTRO Handbook of Radiation Oncology http://www.estroweb.org/estro/book/
Brachytherapy	Radiation Oncologists and Technologists	Recommendations for implementation of high dose rate 192-Ir brachytherapy in developing countries by the Advisory Group of International Atomic Energy Agency Radiotherapy and Oncology 64(3):297-308 (2002)
Core Training	Radiation Technologists	Review of the European Core Curriculum for Radiation Technologists http://www.estroweb.org/ESTRO/upload/pdfs/DK2003FINAL.pdf *Danish* http://www.estroweb.org/ESTRO/upload/pdfs/NL2003FINAL.pdf *Dutch* http://www.estroweb.org/ESTRO/upload/pdfs/EN20Mar2003FINAL.pdf *English* http://www.estroweb.org/ESTRO/upload/pdfs/FIN-CC-Feb2003-FINAL.pdf *Finnish* http://www.estroweb.org/ESTRO/upload/pdfs/FR2003FINAL.pdf *French* http://www.estroweb.org/ESTRO/upload/pdfs/DE2003FINAL.pdf *German* http://www.estroweb.org/ESTRO/upload/pdfs/GR2003FINAL.pdf *Greek* http://www.estroweb.org/ESTRO/upload/pdfs/IT2003FINAL.pdf *Italian* http://www.estroweb.org/ESTRO/upload/pdfs/PT2003FINAL.pdf *Portuguese* http://www.estroweb.org/ESTRO/upload/pdfs/ES2003FINAL.pdf *Spanish* http://www.estroweb.org/ESTRO/upload/pdfs/SE2003FINAL.pdf *Swedish*
Training	Physicists	Guideline for education and training of medical physicists in radiation http://www.estroweb.org/ESTRO/upload/GUIDELINES/CC-MPhys.pdf

17. Palliative Care

Agency	Audience	Resource and Link
IAHPC	Health Care Providers	International Association for Hospital and Palliative Care manual of palliative care. http://www.hospicecare.com/manual/toc-main.html *English*
WHO	Health Care Provider	WHO Journal on issues related to cancer and pain control http://www.whocancerpain.wisc.edu/index.html
NCBI	Policy and Health Care Providers	Disease Control Priorities Project – Disease Control Priorities in Developing Countries: Chap 52-Pain Control for People with Cancer and AIDs

		http://www.ncbi.nlm.nih.gov/books/bv.fcgi?rid=dcp2.chapter.7766
ISNCC	Nurses	Curriculum for Palliative Nursing A core curriculum for a post basic course in palliative nursing © 2003 http://www.isncc.org/lists.asp?table=Publications#Core
ACCP	Health Care Providers	Palliative Support – Fact Sheet ©2003 http://www.path.org/files/RH_palliative_care_fs.pdf *English* http://www.path.org/files/RH_palliative_care_fs_sp.pdf *Spanish* http://www.path.org/files/RH_palliative_care_fs_fr.pdf *French* http://www.path.org/files/RH_palliative_care_fs_r.pdf *Russian*
ACCP	Managers	Supporting women with cancer © 2004 http://www.path.org/files/RH_supporting_women_iid.pdf *French and Spanish*
ASCO	Health Care Providers	http://www.asco.org/portal/site/ASCO/menuitem.5d1b4bac73a9104ce277e89a320041a0/?vgnextoid=b1fbc2931f48d010VgnVCM100000ed730ad1RCRD
ACCP	Managers	Planning and Implementing a Cancer Control Program: Chapter of Palliative Care http://www.path.org/files/RH_accp_mfm_p4.pdf

Chapter 2

BREAST CANCER

SECTION 1: AGENCIES AND SOCIETIES INVOLVED IN BREAST CANCER WORK IN THE MAJORITY WORLD

We have indicated where information was available whether the society or agency had regional representation from the majority world on their board or whether they had branch offices in countries of the majority world

Agency		**Weblink**	
United Nations			
IAEA International Atomic Energy Agency		http://www.iaea.org/	International Atomic Energy Agency P.O. Box 100 Wagramer Strasse 5 A-1400 Vienna, Austria Tel: (+431) 2600-0 Fax: (+431) 2600-7 IAEA Office at the United Nations 1 United Nations Plaza Room DC-1-1155 New York, NY 10017 USA Tel: (001) 212-963-6010 or 6011 Fax: (001) 917-367-4046 IAEA Office in Geneva United Nations Room B 426 Palais des Nations CH-1211 Geneva 10 Switzerland Tel: (+41-22) 917-3632 Fax: (+41-22) 917-0066

PACT Programme of Action for Cancer Treatment		http://www-naweb.iaea.org/pact/	Mr. Massoud Samiei PACT Programme Manager International Atomic Energy Agency P.O. Box 100 Wagramer Strasse 5 A-1400 Vienna, Austria pact@iaea.org
World Health Organization			
WHO : World Health Organization		http://who.int	Avenue Appia 20 1211 Geneva 27 Switzerland Telephone: (+ 41 22) 791 21 11 Facsimile (fax): (+ 41 22) 791 3111 Telex: 415 416 Telegraph: UNISANTE GENEVA
IARC: International Agency for Research in Cancer		http://www.iarc.fr/	IARC 150 Cours Albert-Thomas 69372 Lyon Cedex 08 France Tel +33 (0) 472738485 FAX 33 (0) 472738575
Regional Office for PAHO: PanAmerican Health Organization		http://www.paho.org/	Regional Office for the Americas 525, 23rd Street, N.W. Washington, DC 20037 USA Telephone: +1 202 974 3000 Facsimile: +1 202 974 3663 E-mail: postmaster@paho.org Regional Director: Dr Mirta Roses
Regional Office for Africa		http://www.afro.who.int/	Regional Office for Africa Cite du Djoue, P.O.Box 06 Brazzaville, Congo Telephone: + 242 839 100 / +47 241 39100 Facsimile: + 242 839 501 / +47 241 395018 E-mail: regafro@whoafr.org Regional Director: Dr L. Sambo
Regional Office for South-East Asia		http://www.searo.who.int/	Regional Office for South-East Asia World Health House Indraprastha Estate Mahatama Gandhi Marg New Delhi 110 002 India Telephone: + 91-11-2337 0804

			Facsimile: + 91-11-2337 9507 E-mail: pandeyh@whosea.org
Regional Office for Europe		http://www.euro.who.int/	Regional Director: Dr Samlee Plianbangchang Regional Office for Europe 8, Scherfigsvej DK-2100 Copenhagen 0, Denmark Telephone: + 45 39 171 717 Facsimile: + 45 39 171 818 E-mail: postmaster@euro.who.int
Regional Office for Eastern Mediterranean		http://www.emro.who.int/	Regional Director: Marc Danzon Regional Office for the Eastern Mediterranean Abdul Razzak Al Sanhouri Street, P.O. Box 7608, Nasr City, Cairo 11371, Egypt Telephone: + 202 670 25 35 Facsimile: + 202 670 24 92 or 670 24 94 E-mail: postmaster@emro.who.int Regional Director: Dr Hussein Abdel-Razzak Al Gezairy
Regional Office for Western Pacific		http://www.wpro.who.int/	Regional Office for the Western Pacific P.O. Box 2932 1000 Manila Philippines Telephone: + 63 2 528 8001 E-mail: postmaster@wpro.who.int Regional Director: Dr Shigeru Omi
Governmental Organizations			
CDC: Centres for disease control		http://www.cdc.gov/	Centers for Disease Control and Prevention, 1600 Clifton Rd, Atlanta, GA 30333, U.S.A Tel: (404) 639-3311 / Public Inquiries: (404) 639-3534 / (800) 311-3435
NCI: National Cancer Institute		http://www.cancer.gov/	NCI Public Inquiries Office 6116 Executive Boulevard Room 3036A Bethesda, MD 20892-8322 Tel: 1-800-4-CANCER / (1-800-422-6237)

Nongovernmental organizations			
	Intn org of committees or intn offices		
American Cancer Society (ACS)		http://www.cancer.org/docroot/home/index.asp	Tel: 1-800-ACS-2345 (1-866-228-4327)
EngenderHealth	20 offices in the field, and more than 70% of our staff work in countries across Asia, Africa, and the Americas	http://www.engenderhealth.org/	EngenderHealth 440 Ninth Avenue New York, New York 10001 USA Contact: Jan Bradley, M.A. Tel: (212) 561-8000
Fred Hutchinson Cancer Research Centre	Intl research projects only	http://www.fhcrc.org/	Fred Hutchinson Cancer Research Center P.O. Box 19024 Seattle, WA 98109-1024 Phone: (206) 288-1024 Toll-free: (800) 804-8824 Fax: (206) 288-1025
International Union Against Cancer (UICC)	Yes	http://www.uicc.org	International Union Against Cancer (UICC) 62 route de Frontenex 1207 Geneva Switzerland Tel +41 22 809 1811 Fax + 41 22 809 1810
JHPIEGO, an affiliate of Johns Hopkins University	Yes	http://www.jhpiego.org/	JHPIEGO 1615 Thames Street Baltimore, Maryland 21231 USA Tel: (410) 537-1913
PATH: Programme in advanced technologies in Health	Yes	http://www.path.org/	PATH Alliance coordinating agency 1455 NW Leary Way Seattle, Washington 98107 USA Tel: (206) 285-3500
Susan G. Komer Breast Cancer Foundation	No	http://cms.komen.org/komen/index.htm	5005 LBJ Freeway, Suite 250 Dallas, TX 75244 Telephone: 972-855-1600 Fax: 972-855-1605
International Societies			
American College of Surgeons	No	http://www.facs.org/	633 N St. Claire St. Chicago IL 60611-3211 Tel: (312) 202-5000 Toll free: 1 (800) 621-4114 FAX: (312) 202-5001 Email: postmaster@facs.org

American Society of Breast Disease			
American Society of Breast Surgeons	No	http://www.breastsurgeons.org/	The American Society of Breast Surgeons 5950 Symphony Woods Road Suite 212 Columbia, MD 21044 Tel: 410-992-5470 Toll free 877-992-5470 Fax: 410-992-5472 E-Mail: contact@breastsurgeons.org
American Society of Clinical oncology (ASCO)	No	http://www.asco.org/	American Society of Clinical Oncology 1900 Duke Street, Suite 200 Alexandria, VA 22314 Tel: 703-299-0150 Fax: 703-299-1044 E-mail: asco@asco.org
Association International for Breast Cancer Research	No Fund research without boundaries	http://www.aicr.org.uk/	Phone: 01334 - 477910
Australasian Society for Breast Disease (ASBD)	No	http://www.asbd.org.au/	PO Box 1124 Coorparoo DC Qld 4151 Australia Phone: +61 7 3847 1946 Fax: +61 7 3847 7563 Email: info@asbd.org.au
Breast International Group	No	http://www.breastinternationalgroup.org/default.htm Research group with representation from specific research groups	
Breast Surgery International (BSI)	Yes	http://www.breast-surg-intl.org/	Dr. Gaurav Agarwal MS, DNB, PDC, C-RACS (EndocrSurg) Secretary, BSI Associate Professor Dept. of Endocrine & Breast Surgery Sanjay Gandhi PG Institute of Medical Sciences Raebareli Road, Lucknow - 226 014, INDIA Phone: +91-522-2668700 ext.-2160 Fax: +91-522-2668017 E-mail: gaurav@sgpgi.ac.in, GauravBSI@gmail.com

Cochrane Breast Cancer Group	No	http://www.ctc.usyd.edu.au/cochrane/links/7d_healthP_links.htm	
European Society of Gynecologic Oncology (ESGO)	No	http://www.esgo.org/	17 Rue du Cendrier P.O. Box 1726 CH-1211 Geneva 1 Switzerland Tel: +41 22 906 9150 Fax: +41 22 732 2852 E-mail: info@esgo.org
European Society of mastology (EUSOMA)	No	http://www.eusoma.org/Engx/About/Default.aspx?cont=default	Via del Pratellino, 7 50131 Florence - Italy Tel: +39 055 576.260 Fax: +39 055 5537.4209 E-Mail: secretariat@eusoma.org
International Association for Hospice and Palliative Care	No	http://www.hospicecare.com/	*International Association Hospice and Palliative Care* 5535 Memorial Dr. Suite F - PMB 509 Houston TX 77007 USA Tel: +1 (936) 321-9846 Toll Free +1 (866) 374 2472 Fax +1 (713) 880-2948
International Breast cancer research foundation	No	http://www.ibcrf.org/	The International Breast Cancer Research Foundation 4230 East Towne Boulevard, #173 Madison, WI 53704 Phone: 608.268.3077 FAX: 608.246.3019
International Breast Screening Research Group	No	http://appliedresearch.cancer.gov/ibsn/ Research	Emily Dowling Program Analyst phone: (301) 594-6654 fax: (301) 435-3710 e-mail: dowlinge@mail.nih.gov Applied Research Program Division of Cancer Control and Population Sciences National Cancer Institute Executive Plaza North, Room 4111 6130 Executive Blvd., MSC 7344 Bethesda, MD 20892-7344
International Gynecologic Cancer Society	Yes	http://www.igcs.org/	IGCS PO Box 6387 Louisville KY 40206 USA Tel: 1 (502) 891.4575 FAX 1 (502) 891.4576
International Network for Cancer Treatment and Research (INCTR)	No	http://www.inctr.org/	INCTR At the Institut Pasteur Rue Engeland 642 Brussels B-1180 Belgium
International Society of Breast Pathology (ISBP)	No	http://www.isbp.info/	Office of the Secretary International Society of Breast Pathology Department of Pathology

			Memorial Sloan-Kettering 1275 York Ave. New York, NY 10021 Phone: (212) 639-5905 Fax: (212) 717-3203 E-mail: tanl@mskcc.org
International Society for Nurses in Cancer Care (ISNCC)	Not clear	http://www.isncc.org/	108 Chestergate Macclesfield Cheshire SK11 6DU United Kingdom Tel/Fax: +44 162 566 9588 Email: secretariat@isncc.org
Middle East Cancer Consortium	No	http://mecc.cancer.gov/	
Senologic International Society	Yes	http://www.sisbreast.org/	rorda@post.tau.ac.il
Society of Gynecologic Oncologists (SGO)	No	http://www.sgo.org/	
Society of Surgical Oncology	No	http://www.surgonc.org/	
World Society for Breast Health (WSBH)		http://www.wsbh.org/ Based on societies that join this society	K&M Congress Ltd. Ms Katalin Mátray H-1064 Budapest, Podmaniczky u. 75. Phone: +36-1-3012000, Fax: +36-1-3012001 wsbh@kmcongress.com

SECTION 2 : PUBLISHED RESEARCH ON BREAST CANCER IN THE CARIBBEAN, MEXICO, CENTRAL AND SOUTH AMERICA

The search terms were "breast cancer" and "control" and "program" in MEDLINE and GOOGLE (1716 hits: 1958-2006) 1Nov2006. Information is categorized by country. Where an abstract was available, this was included.

Country	Reference
Latin America	Solé Barja C. Mamocintigrafía / Mammoscintigraphy. Rev. Méd. Clín. Condes. 2002;13(1):26-29 Mammography is the diagnostic method with the greatest usefulness, both in screening and in diagnosing breast cancer. However, although mammography is a highly sensitive technique, it is frequently incapable od differentiating malignant lesions from benign ones, having this method a positive predictive value (PPV) that ranges between 10 percent and 40 percent. This PPV causes a large number of unnecessary breast biopsies to be performed on bening lesions. Furthermore, in joung women, fibrocystic disease, dense breat or evaluation

	after biopsy, surgery or Radiotherapy, the performance of mammography is much lower and the diagnosis of the cancer is occacionally impossible. Bearing in mind all these limitations, it becomes clear the importance of having available a complementary diagnostic procedure that allows the PPV of mammography to be improved and that completes the study of patients who are difficult to evaluate by way of mammography. It has been suggest that 99m Tc - MiBi Scintimammography, used as a complementary technique to mammography, is a useful test in the examination of patients with suspected breast cancer. The adoption of a joint mammography - Scintimammography diagnostic protocol could considerably reduce the number of biopsies perfomed in patients with lesion of low or indeterminate mammographic suspicion of malignanacy (BIRADS 3, - BIRADS 4). Larger series will be necessary to determine the definitive value of this protocol, which has been drawn up to select those patients with suspected breast cancer in whom a biopsy of the lesion should be performed
	Medina V, Margarita R; Hincapie Celis, Cecilia; Guevara Pardo, Gonzálo; Perry Perry, Fernándo; Ramos Vargas, Juan. Cancer de seno: historia de enfermedad de mujeres consultantes al Instituto de Cancerología / Breat cancer: history of disease of women consultants to the Institute of Cancerology. Santa Fe de Bogotá; Instituto Nacional de Salud; jun. 1999. 180
	Freitas Júnior R, Conti RC. Quimioterapia do câncer de mama. Ja é chegada a hora? / Chemioteapy of breat cancer. Has the time come? Femina; 1993;21(11):1181-4
	Llanos G, Hoffenberg LM. Detection of breast cancer: Implications for Latin América and the Caribbean. Washington, D.C; Pan Américan Health Organization; Nov. 1992. 9 p. ilus. (PAHO. Informational Synopsis, 1/92). The recommendation of the Health Promotion Program of the Pan Américan Health Organization is that in Latina América "self-examination should be initiated before de age of 35,"and thus the efforts should be directed toward education. In general, physicians and nurses must be well trained to carry out a good physical examination of the breast each time that the woman visits a clinic. And the task of educating women about self-examinations should be a routine part of programs in institutions of health, education, and the workplace, etc. Mammography, given its high cost in our Region, should not be utilized in mass programs, but rather should be reserved as a procedure to follow-up high-risk women, or for those with suspected pathology
	Espinoz H, Ellertson C, García S, Schiavon R, Langer A. Medicamentos para la interrupción de la gestación: una revisión de la literatura y sus posibles implicaciones para México América Latina / Medical methods for pregnancy termination. A review of literature and its potential role in Mexico and Latin America. Gac. méd. Méx. 2002;138(4):347-356 In this document, we review the relevant aspects of the different medical methods of abortion. We describe the principal medical regimens currently used in North America, Europe, and a growing number of developing countries. We also describe specific treatment regimens (which usually involve a combination of two drugs), physiological methods of action, potential side

	effects and complications, method requirements, including follow-up visits, any existing contraindication, and acceptability of these methods among patients. Finally, we comment on the potential role of medical abortion in Mexico and throughout Latin America.
	Peña-Rosas JP, Rickard, S, Cho SS. Salvado de trigo y cáncer de mama: revisitando la hipótesis del estrógeno / Wheat bran and breast cancer: revisiting the estrogen hypothesis. Arch. latinoam. nutr. 1999;49(4):309-317 Breast cancer is the most relevant form of cancer among women in Latin America. Many studies have evaluated the hormonal mechanisms involved in mammary carcinogenesis, although new focus is aimed towards factors that can potentially be used individually to reduce risk. Wheat bran seems to show a consistent protective effect in mammary carcinogenesis. Wheat bran, besides high level of insoluble fiber, also contains phytic acid and lignins, phytochemicals that have shown to inhibit in vitro and in vivo growth of mammary cancer. The protective effect of wheat bran in breast carcinogenesis is greatest at the promotional phase and when supplemented to a high fat diet. Doses of wheat bran in the 9-12 range have been consistently protective and the inconsistencies observed at higher doses may be dependent on the animal model used. This review examines the protective role of wheat bran in the development of breast cancer and the possible mechanisms involved.
	Bosetti C, Malvezzi M, Chatenoud L, Negri E, Levi F, La Vecchia C. Trends in cancer mortality in the Americas, 1970-2000. Ann Oncol 2005;16(3):489-511 BACKGROUND: Data and statistics on cancer mortality over the last decades are available for most developed countries, while they are more difficult to obtain, in a standardized and comparable format, for countries of Latin America. PATIENTS AND METHODS: Age standardized (world population) mortality rates around the year 2000, derived from the WHO database, are presented for 14 selected cancers and total cancer in 10 countries of Latin America, plus, for comparative purposes, Canada and the USA. Trends in mortality are also given over the period 1970-2000. RESULTS: In 2000, the highest total cancer mortality for males was observed in Argentina and Chile, with rates comparable to those of Canada and the USA, i.e. about 155/100,000. For women, Chile and Cuba had the highest rates in Latin America (114 and 103/100,000, respectively), again comparable to those of North America (around 105/100,000). These reflect the comparatively high mortality from cancer of the stomach (for Chile), lung and intestines (for Argentina) in men, and of stomach and uterus (for Chile), intestines and lung (for Cuba) in women. Colombia, Ecuador and Mexico had the lowest total cancer mortality for men, due to low mortality from stomach, colorectal and lung cancer. For women, the lowest rates were in Brazil and Puerto Rico, reflecting their low stomach and cervical cancer rates. In Argentina, Chile, Colombia, Costa Rica and Venezuela cancer mortality rates tended to decline, particularly in men. Rates were stable in Ecuador and Puerto Rico, and were increasing in Mexico and Cuba. CONCLUSIONS: Mortality from some common cancers (including colorectal and lung) is still low in Latin America compared with Canada and the USA, and decreasing trends have been observed in the last decades for some cancer

	sites (including stomach, uterus, lung and other tobacco-related cancers) in several countries. However, mortality from female lung and breast cancers has been increasing in most countries of Latin America, and several countries still show an extremely elevated mortality from cancer of the cervix. Selected neoplasms amenable to treatment, including testis and leukemias, also show unsatisfactory trends in Latin America.
	Robles S, Galanis E. Breast cancer in Latin America and the Caribbean. Rev. panam. salud pública 2002;11(3):178-185 As recently as two decades ago breast cancer was not a significant public health concern in Latin America and the Caribbean (LAC). However, mortality rates from breast cancer have been increasing for at least 40 years in most LAC countries. Socioeconomic development and consequent changes in reproductive behaviors over the past 50 years are thought to have contributed to the increased risk of breast cancer. Socioeconomic development has also increased women's health awareness and therefore the demand for quality services. In industrialized countries, screening and widely available, high-quality treatment protocols are being implemented as the main strategy for breast cancer control. Studies show that out of three available screening methods (mammography, clinical breast examination, and breast self-examination), only mammography for women 50-69 years of age has been effective at reducing mortality, and has done so by an estimated 23%. While there is much controversy about the benefits and cost-effectiveness of mammography screening for women aged 40-49, some countries, including Australia, the United States of America, and four European nations, recommend that physicians assess the need for it on an individual basis. A survey that we conducted of LAC countries shows that most of their breast cancer screening policies are not justified by available scientific evidence. Moreover, as seen by relatively high mortality/incidence ratios, breast cancer cases are not being adequately managed in many LAC countries. Before further developing screening programs, these countries need to evaluate the feasibility of designing and implementing appropriate treatment guidelines and providing wide access to diagnostic and treatment services. Given the relevance of breast cancer in Latin America and the Caribbean today, it is crucial that both women and health care providers have access to up-to-date information on which to base their decisions
	Anderson BO. Breast healthcare and cancer control in limited-resource countries: a framework for change. Nature Clinical Practice Oncology 2006; 3: 4-5 Breast cancer is the most common cause of cancer-related death among women around the globe. Each year, breast cancer is newly diagnosed in more than 1.1 million women, and these cases represent more than 10% of all new cancer cases. With more than 410,000 deaths each year, breast cancer accounts for over 1.6% of all female deaths worldwide.Breast cancer is already an urgent public health problem in high-resource regions, and is becoming an increasingly urgent problem in low-resource regions, where incidence rates have been increasing by up to 5% per year.Low-resource countries have

	generally not identified cancer as a priority healthcare issue because infectious disease is the predominant public health threat in such settings; however, resources are inevitably spent on cancer treatment when patients seek medical care for what is typically advanced-stage disease. Furthermore, as life expectancy in these countries increases through the control of communicable disease, cancer becomes an increasing problem. Obstacles to improving cancer care arise from multiple sources, including deficits in public knowledge and awareness, social and cultural barriers, challenges in organizing healthcare, and insufficient resources. http://www.nature.com/ncponc/journal/v3/n1/pdf/ncponc0397.pdf
	Llanos G. Detection of breast cancer: Implications for Latin America and the Caribbean. Washington, D.C; Pan American Health Organization. Health Promotion Program; Nov. 1992. 9 p. (Informational Synopsis, 1/92).
Argentina	Matos EL, et al. Breast cancer in Argentian: case-control study with special reference to meat-eating habits. Neoplasma 38;357-366,1991
	Maria Ines Marchegiani de Ucke, UICC July2006 Breast Cancer Screening Program Objective: In Argentina, the most common cancer in women is breast cancer. The value of mammographic screening in reducing breast cancer mortality and morbidity has been investigated and proven over many years. Population-based screening has demonstrated that many breast cancers detected in the preclinical phase could be successfully treated. Methods: LALCEC mobile mammography unit has begun operating in 1999. The mammogram and clinical examination are performed in the mobile unit, which travels from one place to another, particularly visiting towns with no mammography facility. At each location, the screening is performed on asymptomatic women aged 40-65 pre-registered. The unit stays in each town for a week and travels to the next scheduled place over the weekend, in order to start work again on Monday. Patients diagnosed with breast cancer symptoms are closely monitored until final results and the information from the pathologist are obtained. This Program also covers the operation and treatment of the patient. Results: Since the launching of this Program, more than 66.600 mammograms were provided free of charge to women who would otherwise not likely have received mammography screening. Of the women reached, the majority were illiterate and all of them were low-income and uninsured, 1.363 diagnostic procedures were performed and breast cancer was diagnosed in 324 women. This epidemiological research program is quite new in Argentina and allows us to gather and analyze information regarding the incidence of breast cancer in our Argentina and will provide a scientific basis for breast cancer prevention.
	Frahm I. National HER2 testing program for breast cancer patients in Argentina. *Journal of Clinical Oncology*, 2006 ASCO Annual Meeting Proceedings (Post-Meeting Edition).2006; 24(18S): 10566 Background: In Argentina, before 2003 few pathologists performed HER2 testing, using different non-standardized Inmuno-Histo-Chemical (IHC) methods with dubious and non-reproducible results and also leaving some parts of the country without HER2 diagnosis Objective: HER2 has a key role in breast cancer management, so the aim of the study was to settle a National

	HER2 testing Program to permit access to standardized HER2 detection all over the country, and whenever possible, to determine hormonal receptors. Methods: In August 2003, 13 pathologists formed a cooperative group and created a national framework to train and set HER2 diagnostic centres in each country region. A coordinator responsible for coaching and evaluating centres and two technical consultants in charge of quality control and technique standardization were designated. In February 2004, the program was launched. Tumors were received from 82 oncologists and breast surgeons, using a private courier created "ad hoc". HER2 was analyzed by IHC test between February 2004 and November 2005 and performed using policlonal antibody anti Her 2 (DAKO), microwave antigenic recovery, detection system EnVision (Dako) and developed with diaminobenzidine. Results were interpreted as HercepTest guidelines. ER/PR were screened by IHC analyses. Results: 2285 HER2 tests were performed: HER2 was over-expressed (score 3+) in 18% of tumors (408). 136 (6%) samples were score 2+, 407 (18%) score 1+ and 1334 (58%) score 0. In 1532/2285 (67%) of tumor specimens ER and PR status could be determined. Conclusions: Founding HER2 National Program allowed access to HER2 testing all over the country with a standardized and reproducible technique. HER2 prevalence in our sample (18%) is similar to those previously published. Although international algorithms recommend FISH assay to HER2 2+ tumors, our Program can not afford it. ER/PR expression were decreased significantly in HER2 3+ vs. HER2 - tumors: 53% vs. 64%: $p = 0.002$. HER2 3+ were associated with higher levels ER/PR: 38% vs. 24% in HER2 - tumors ($p < 0.001$). http://meeting.jco.org/cgi/content/abstract/24/18_suppl/10566
	Schwartsmann G. Breast Cancer in South America: Challenges to Improve Early Detection and Medical Management of a Public Health Problem From the Comprehensive Cancer Center, The Lutheran University of Brazil, and Federal University of Rio Grande do Sul, Porto Alegre, Brazil. http://www.jco.org/cgi/content/full/19/suppl_1/118s
	Bruno S, Puerot VL et al. Phase II trial of weekly IV vinorelbine as a single agent in first-line advanced breast cancer chemotherapy: The Latin-American experience Am j Clin Oncol 5:392-396,1995
	Iscovich JM, Iscovich RB, Howe G, Shiboski S, Kaldor JM. A case–control study of diet and breast cancer in Argentina. Int J Cancer 1989; 44: 770–776 A case-control study of breast cancer was carried out in La Plata, Argentina, where the incidence of the disease is comparable to the highest rates recorded worldwide. One hundred and fifty incident cases were identified through major hospitals. For each case, a hospital control, matched by age and hospital, and a neighbourhood control, matched by residential area and age, were also chosen. Cases and controls were interviewed to obtain information on past diet, as well as demographic and socio-economic characteristics, reproductive and menstrual history and other potential breast-cancer risk factors. The dietary information was obtained from questions on the consumption of specific food items and information on portion sizes from an earlier study was used to estimate intake of calories and selected nutrients. There was a substantial excess energy intake among cases as compared to both control groups, which was present across all 3 major macronutrients which contribute to total

	calories. Among the food groups, the consumption of eggs was a risk factor for breast cancer, and whole-milk products and green leafy vegetables were protective. After adjusting for the calorie difference in multivariate statistical analyses of nutrients, fibre and beta-carotene consumption were weakly protective. The results are discussed with reference to possible methodological difficulties and previous studies of diet and breast cancer.
	ARREDONDO A, LOCKETT LY, ICAZA E. Cost of diseases in Brazil: breast cancer, enteritis, cardiac valve disease and bronchopneumonia. *Rev. Saúde Pública*, Oct. 1995;29(5):349-354. The results from the need to develop methodologies for performing cost analysis in developing countries, principally in the region of Latin America, were studied. It, furthermore, serves to generate knowledge from an economic evaluation in order to support decision-making related to the organization of health systems, particularly in the efficient use of resources which are allocated for the provision of medical services. Two chronic diseases (breast cancer and cardiac valve disease) and two infections (enteritis and bronchopneumonia) were selected for the study. The results recommend the use of a valid methodology for economic cost analysis of any disease to be studied and the use of this information in the decision-making process.
Brazil	de Freitas Junior R, de Oliveira EL,Marinho ER, Zampronha RA, Pereira RJ, Soares FA. Knowledge on screening and diagnosis of breast cancer among gynecologists in Goias State (Brazil). Rev Assoc Med Bras 2003;Jul-Sep,49(3):312-6 OBJECTIVES: To evaluate the knowledge level on the screening and diagnosis of breast cancer among the gynecologists of the State of Goias, Brazil. METHODS: Questionnaires containing professional information and questions on breast cancer screening were posted for all the 427 gynecologists associated to the Goias Society of Gynecology and Obstetrics, between May and July of 1999. RESULTS: Of the 427 questionnaires, 26 (6%) were returned because incorrect mailing address. Of the 401 doctors who received the questionnaire, 85 (21%) answered and returned them back. Of these, 28% were female; the average of the profession time was of 17 years. The medical residence was the highest title level for 70%. The average age of the doctors was 44 years. The rates of correct answers were: 94% for the knowledge of the most frequent sign of breast cancer, 75% for the best method for screening, 88% for the period of when the mammography begins, 93% for the periodicity of the mammography after the 50 years and 83% about the indication of the complementary ultrasound. The doctors who have studied in a program of medical residence was the only factor that influenced the rate of correct answers, if compared to those that did not cursed it. The professional's gender, the Title in Gynecology and Obstetrics Specialty (TEGO) holders and the city of work did not influence the rates of correct answers. CONCLUSION: The gynecologists of the State of Goias who answered the questionnaire have a good knowledge on the screening and diagnosis of breast cancer. Medical residence was the single factor that influenced the rate of correct answers.
	Pinottija , Barros ACSD, Hegg R. Zeferino LC. Breast disease 1995, vol. 8, n°3, pp. 243-250 Breast cancer is a very important health problem in developing countries,

	where its incidence has increased in the past decades. Mortality rates due to breast cancer have also increased, and the main reason for this is late diagnosis. Organizing programs for early breast cancer detection is possible with simple resources. We propose a set of tiered interventions, stratified by levels of complexity. Level 1 = identification of abnormal breast by health professionals ; level 2 = medical assistance to women whose breasts are considered abnormal, to diagnose and treat benign diseases and recognize suspected cases of cancer ; level 3 = management of women with suspected or diagnosed breast cancer by a multidisciplinary team. http://cat.inist.fr/?aModele=afficheN&cpsidt=3546944
	Pazos C et al. Phase 2 study of doxorubicin/Taxol in metastatic breast cancer: Argentine Multicenter Taxol Group. Breast Cancer Res Treat 1999;55;91-96
	Schwartsmann G et al. A phase 2 study of doxorubicin/paclitaxel plus G-CSF for metastatic breast cancer. Oncology 1997;11:24-29
	Murad AM et al. Gemcitabine and paclitaxel as salvage therapy in metastatic breast cancer. Oncology 2001;15 (supp 3):25-27
	Murad AM et al. Phase 2 trial of paclitaxel and ifosfamide as salvage treatment in metastatic breast cancer. Breast Can Res Treat 1997;45:47-53
	Modeste NN, Barriers to early detection of breast cancer among women of carribbean population. PAHJ mar1999;5(3):152-6 The purpose of this descriptive study was to identify and describe barriers to early detection of breast cancer, as well as current breast cancer screening behaviors and attitudes regarding the disease, among women aged 20 and older on the Caribbean island of Tobago. Tobago is the smaller of the two islands that make up the nation of Trinidad and Tobago. Between February and June 1996, 265 women fitting the age criteria completed a structured survey questionnaire. Women of Agrican descent made up 89 per cent of the respondents. In terms of age, 48 per cent of those surveyed were between 20 and 39, 40 per cent were between 40 and 59, and 12 per cent were 60 or older. Barriers to early detection identified were a low level of breast self-examination, infrequent clinical breast examinations as part of regular care, unavailability of mammography services on Tobago, cost of screening, and difficulty of traveling to Trinidad for mammography. Furthermore, only a minority of the study participants had ever attended early detection or public awareness programs. The results were nearly the same for individuals with a family history of breast cancer, who would have a higher risk of occurrence of the disease. In addition, the majority of the respondents reported what can be considered a cultural barrier to early detection practices, a belief that no matter what they did, if they were to get breast cancer, they would get it. The authors recommend that mammography services be made available on Tobago. The authors also intend to use the findings to help develop an appropriate, culturally sensitive breast cancer awareness and early detection program for women on the island
	Campos B, Díez O, Alvarez C, Palma L, Domènech M, Balmaña J, Sanz J, Ramírez A, Alonso C, Carvallo P, Baiget M. Análisis del haplotipo en portadores de la mutación 6857delAA en el gen BRCA2 en 4 familias con cáncer de mama u ovario hereditario. [Haplotype of the BRCA2 6857delAA

	mutation in 4 families with breast/ovarian cancer]. Med Clin (Barc);123(14):543-5, 2004 Oct 23. BACKGROUND AND OBJECTIVE: It is estimated that 5-10% of all breast cancers are hereditary, mainly are due to germline mutations in the BRCA1 and BRCA2 genes. PATIENTS AND METHOD: A BRCA2 screening was carried out in familial breast/ovarian cancer at two centres in Spain and Chile. The 6857delAA mutation was identified in 3 Spanish families and one Chilean, all of them with Spanish ancestors. The BRCA2 haplotype of the 6857delAA carriers was analyzed using five microsatellite markers flanking the BRCA2 gene, spanning a region of 6 cM: cen-D13S260, D13S1698, (BRCA2), D13S171, D13S310 and D13S267-tel. RESULTS: Two families shared the allelic variants of the 5 microsatellites studied. Markers D13S260 and D13S267 differed in one allele in two families, respectively. The defined haplotype was absent in non-carriers from these families, and was not detected in 100 control chromosomes without the mutation. CONCLUSIONS: Our results suggest the existence of a common ancestry with the mutation originating in the Northeast of Spain. Given the migratory movements from Spain to Latin America, the screening of recurrent Spanish mutations can be useful in establishing a more rational and cost-effective analysis in such populations.
Caribbean	Atalah E et al. Breast cancer risk factors in women in Santiago, Chile. Rev Med Chil 2:137-143,2000
Chile	Schencke M et al. Attitude and behavior regarding breast self examination in health professionals in Chile. Bol Oficina Sanit panam 114;317-325,1993
	Armijo R. The epidemiology of cancer in Chile Natl Ca Inst Mono 1979;Nov 53, 115-8
	Arriagada R, Rutqvist LE et al. Postmastectomy radiotherapy: Randomized trials. Semin Radiat Oncol. 3:275-286,1999
	Arriagada R, Rutqvist LE. Adequate locoregional treatment for early breast cancer prevents secondary dissemination. J Clin Oncology 12;2869-2878,1995
	Olaya-Contreras P, Pierre B, Lazcano-Ponce E *et al.* Reproductive risk factors associated with breast cancer in Columbian women. *Rev. Saúde Pública*, June 1999, vol.33, no.3, p.237-245. ISSN 0034-8910. INTRODUCTION: As of 1992, breast cancer has been the second cause of death in Columbian women, with a rising trend in mortality due to this type of neoplasm (average annual rate 4.5*/100.000 inhabitants). Information about potential risk factors for breast cancer in Latin American countries is scarce. The objectives of the project were to test the breastfeeding protection against breast cancer and to establish the reproductive factors associated with breast cancer in Columbia. METHODS: A hospital case-control study was carried out from July 1995 to March 1996 in Bogotá, Columbia, using paring by age groups. The study population consisted of 171 histopathologically confirmed cases and 171 controls. Reproductive history and sociodemographic data were collected through a questionnaire, and logistic regression models were used for statistical analysis of the data. RESULTS: The following associated factors were found as principal results: nuli-parousness as compared with women with over 3 children (OR=3.35 CI 1.40-8.0), age at first birth (OR=1.83 CI 0.70-4.80), breast cancer history, breastfeeding the first child (OR=0.09 CI 0.01-

	0.64 for 1-11 months) and with a highly significant trend for accumulated breastfeeding above 24 months (p=0.001). CONCLUSIONS: This study indicates the importance of focusing on the promotion of prolonged breastfeeding by women identified as being at higher risk, and confirms that socio-economic level can determine life styles and reproductive events among women (such as breastfeeding time); this could explain the increase in breast cancer mortality in Latin American countries, similar to that in developed countries in terms of fertility and risk factors for breast cancer. The epidemiological information produced by this study will be useful for planning and carrying out early diagnosis and treatment of breast cancer in women identified as being at high risk of this disease.
	Olaya-Contresras P et al. Organochloride exposure and breast cancer risk in Colombian women. Cad Saude Publica 14;125-132, 1998 (S3)
	Fernandez L, Buch ML, Molina A, Carabelloso M, Gausioso R, Lage A. Risk factors in mass screening for breast cancer, multivariate analysis of data from the Cuban diagnosis pilot study. Neoplasma 1986 33(4) 535-41 The evolution of mammography has provided possibilities for mass screening programs. Early diagnosis is considered the most important factor in reducing the breast cancer mortality but the mass screening is very expensive if we include all female population. In this paper we show the results of an early diagnosis pilot study with a multivariate data analysis. Data concerning risk factors (age, age at menarche, menopause, parity, age at first childbirth, lactation, abortions and previous benign breast disease) were recorded in 438 patients with breast carcinoma and 1750 patients with benign breast diseases diagnosed in the Early Diagnosis Pilot Program at the National Institute of Oncology and Radiobiology in Cuba. A group of 449 healthy women living in Havana City was also studied. Age and age at first childbirth were the major factor considered. Multivariate data analysis allowed to build stratification trees identifying subgroups with different breast cancer incidence. The usefulness of these stratifications for screening with optimal coverage, sufficiency and efficacy, is discussed.
Columbia	Guarner J, Valdivieso E, Quintana A, Frias M. CA 15.3 in breast cancer: Comparison of two assays and validation in a mexican population. Arch. med. res;28(4):523-6, dec. 1997. Ca 15.3 is a tumor marker used for breat carcinoma, since one epitope is an antigen present in milk fat globules. Serum from 171 patients with breast cancer upon initial presentation was studied for Ca 15.3. In the first 72 cases, the authors compared RIA vs. ELISA using a simple linear regression. On the following 99, only ELISA was performed. With all 171 patients, a clinical association between Ca 15.3 mesurement and age, stage and hormone receptors was carried out. Correlation coefficient between RIA and ELISA was 0.85. Of 104 patients below 50 years of age, 88 had normal Ca 15.3 and 16, elevated; 67 were older than 50 years, 46 had normal Ca 15.3 and 21, elevated (p=0.022). Ca 15.3 was elevated in 11 percent of patients with clinical stages I/II, and 89 percent in stages III/IV (p=0.0001). The association of Ca 15.3 with hormone receptors was not significant. In conclusion, ELISA and RIA measure Ca 15.3 with comparable results, the first method has the advantage of not using

	radioactivity. The authors found higher probability of elevated Ca 15.3 in older patients and in those with advanced disease(AU).
	Cervantes MG, Torrecillas L, Erazo Valle A. Estudio fase II de docetaxel en pacientes con cáncer de mama avanzado sin tratamiento previo con quimioterapia citotóxica / Phase II study of docetaxel in patients with advance breat cancer without previous treatment and cytotoxic chemotherapy. Rev. Inst. Nac. Cancerol. (Méx.);43(1):14-20, ene.-mar. 1997 Objetivo: Investigar la respuesta y seguridad de docetaxel como terapia de primera línea en cáncer metastásico de mama. Material y métodos: De marzo a octubre de 1994 se incluyeron 16 pacientes con cáncer mamario metastásico; el promedio de edad fue de 46 años y el estado funcional de 0-1; seis con quimioterapia adyuvante; las metástasis más frecuentes fueron a partes blandas, pulmón y huesos. El tratamiento consistió en docetaxel 100 mg x my de superficie corporal cada tes semanas con premedicación a base de cetirizina más prednisona. Catorce casos fueron evaluables para respuesta y 16 para toxicidad (75 ciclos). Resultados: Cinco pacientes tuvieron respuestas completas y cuatro parciales para un total de nueve (66 por ciento), con una supervivencia actuarial a un año del 85 por ciento. Toxicidad: Las reacciones más frecuentes neutropenia grado 3-4 en el 18.6 por ciento de los ciclos, neutropenial febril en 2.6 por ciento, rash alérgico en dos casos y anafilaxia en una. También se observó edema con incremento de peso en seis casos y en otros tres el edema fue leve. Hubo neuropatía grado 1 en cuatro casos y grado 2 en dos pacientes. Cinco mujeres presentaron piel seca con descamación y tres enfermas exfoliación. Tres pacientes presentaron onicólisis. Se requirió ajuste de dosis en siete ciclos. Conclusiones: Nuestros resultados sugieren la gran respuesta a docetaxel como terapia de primera línea en cáncer mamario metastásico; la toxicidad más frecuente y limitante en la neutropenia y la retención de líquidos.
Cuba	Martinez Abundis G, Cano Rios P, Gonzalez Hernandez S, Rosales Hernandez FJ. Predisposing factors to breast cancer in the Region Langunera (Mexico). Ginecol Obstet Mex 2004;Oct72,525-30 OBJECTIVE: To identify the presence and frequency of various predispose factors of breast cancer in the Region Lagunera (Mexico). PATIENTS AND METHODS: 38 women with breast cancer (Group A, cases) and 24 women without breast pathology (Group B, controls) were analyzed; throughout a questionnaire the variables that have been described as predisposition factors were researched. Group A included patients from the Instituto Mexicano del Seguro Social, Speciality Hospital # 71, Oncology Department in Torreon, Coahuila, from May 1st to October 31st of 1999. At the same time 24 women (Group B), who attended to have an ultrasound and/or a mammography practice in a private clinic in the same city, were polled having a normal result. The means of the two treatments were compared using the SAS program version 6.3. RESULTS: The following variables showed significant difference: mother and father family background with cancer p=0.032; previous breast pathology p=0.0032; hormone consumption p=0.0289; lactation p=0.038 and time of lactation p=0.036. CONCLUSION: Overweight, obesity, mother and father family background with cancer, previous breast pathology background,

	period of consuming hormone, lactation and lactation period had significance in this study.
	Ortega-Altamirano D, Lopez-Carrillo L, Lopez-Cervantes M. Strategies for teaching self-examination of the breast to women in reproductive age. Salud Publica mex 2000 Jan-Feb 42(1) 17-25 OBJECTIVE: To develop an effective strategy to inform Mexican women between 12 and 47 years of age about breast cancer (BC) and train them to perform breast self-examination (BSE). MATERIAL AND METHODS: Between April, 1996 and July, 1998, two different strategies to teach BSE were designed and evaluated in Cuernavaca, State of Morelos, Mexico. These strategies included teaching materials and were based on opinions of women participating in the first stage of this study. Both strategies consisted of the presentation of a leaflet and a video. The first strategy was delivered by a public health nurse in charge of leading the session. The second one was presented by a BC survivor. This second strategy included slides and silicon breast models. These two strategies were then compared to a third one, consisting of a primary care nurse handling out a leaflet and showing a video, based on Health Secretariat's guidelines. In total, 149 women were trained. They were randomly assigned to any one of these three strategies. The effectiveness of the teaching strategies was determined by assessing the changes in the women's knowledge of BC and BSE, as well as in their ability to identify the largest number of lumps on a natural size silicon breast, before and after training. Statistical analysis included Student's t test, variance analysis, McNemar's chi 2, Pearson's chi 2, and multiple linear regression. RESULTS: With all three strategies, there was an increase of approximately 30% in women's knowledge of BC and BSE as well as in their ability to detect lumps. Although at the beginning of the training only one out of every 20 women were able to identify more than three lumps in the silicon model, by the end between 3 and 4 of every 10 women were able to do this, with values of $p < 0.05$. Some factors determine women's learning of both BSE and information about BC as well as their ability to identify lumps. CONCLUSIONS: Teaching BSE with any of the strategies evaluated could be included in an integral program to educate Mexican women on breast cancer prevention and early detection. The appropriate and monthly practice of BSE is linked both to a decrease in the amount of time elapsing between the identification of suspect signs and the demand for medical care, such as requesting a clinical breast examination, which entails identifying small tumors when BC is present.
	Sanchez Ayendez M, Suarez-Perez E, Vazquez MO, Velez-Almodovar H, Nazario CM. Knowledge and beliefs of breast cancer among elderly women in Puerto Rico. Puerto Rico Health Sci 2001;Dec 20(4):351-9 This is the first national study of breast-cancer knowledge, beliefs, and early detection practices among elderly women (65+) in Puerto Rico. Cancer breast examination (CBE) was the most common early detection practice, followed by the mammogram, with breast self exam (BSE) a distant third. The primary reasons most often cited for never having a mammogram related to both personal and external factors: not having symptoms, negligence or forgetfulness, and not having a physician's referral. No statistically significant

	difference ($p < 0.05$) was found between knowledge and early detection practices. Conversely, beliefs had an impact on preventive behavior. Those who had less misconceptions were most likely to have had a CBE or a mammogram. Bivariate analysis demonstrated that age was associated with performing a BSE once or twice monthly, ever having a mammogram, and having a mammogram in the past two years. A higher socioeconomic status was associated to performing BSE and ever having had a mammogram. Education correlated positively to ever having a mammogram or having a mammogram in the two years prior to the interview. Factors that explained compliance with a mammogram in the last two years included referral from a physician, owning a car, and receiving information after menopause on breast cancer from a health care provider. A gynecological visit increased the probability of having had a mammogram during the last two years. Logistic regression determined that a referral from a physician was the most important factor for mammogram compliance when a combination of variables were considered.
Mexico	Oliver-Vazquez M, Sanchez-Ayendez M, Suarez-Perez E, Velez-Almodovar H. Planning a breast cancer health promotion. Qualitative and quantitative data on Puerto Rican elderly women. Prom Edu 1999;Dec 6(4): 16-9,44,54 http://heapro.oxfordjournals.org/cgi/reprint/17/1/3
	Nazario MC, Figueroa-Vallés N, Rosario R. Breast Cancer Patterns and Lifetime Risk of Developing Breast Cancer among Puerto Rican Females. PRHSJ Vol 19 No. 1, March 2000, 7-13.
	Suárez E, Sánchez-Ayéndez M, Oliver-Vázquez M, Almodóvar HV, Rosario-Rosado R, Nazario-Delgado C. Knowledge and Beliefs of Breast Cancer Among Elderly Puerto Rican Women: Validation Process of Scales. PRHSJ 1998, Vol 17, 365-374.
	Walter JP. Outcome of stage 1 carcinoma of the breast at the University hospital of the West Indies (1982-1988). West Indies Med j 1994;43(4):127-129
Puerto Rico	Modeste NN, Caleb-Drayton VL, Montgomery S. Barriers to early detection of breast cancer among women in a Caribbean population . Rev Panam Salud Publica vol.5 n.3 Washington Mar. 1999 The purpose of this descriptive study was to identify and describe barriers to early detection of breast cancer, as well as current breast cancer screening behaviors and attitudes regarding the disease, among women aged 20 and older on the Caribbean island of Tobago. Tobago is the smaller of the two islands that make up the nation of Trinidad and Tobago. Between Febru ary and June 1996, 265 women fitting the age criteria completed a structured survey questionnaire. Women of African descent made up 89% of the respondents. In terms of age, 48% of those surveyed were between 20 and 39, 40% were between 40 and 59, and 12% were 60 or older. Barriers to early detection identified were a low level of breast self-examination, infrequent clinical breast examinations as part of regular care, unavailability of mammography services on Tobago, cost of screening, and difficulty of traveling to Trinidad for mammography. Furthermore, only a minority of the study participants had ever attended early detection or publi c awareness programs. The results were nearly the same for individuals with a family history of breast cancer, who would

	have a higher risk of occurrence of the disease. In addition, the majority of the respondents reported what can be considered a cultural barrier to early detection practices, a belief that no matter what they did, if they were to get breast cancer, they would get it. The authors recommend that mammography services be made available on Tobago. The authors also intend to use the findings to help develop an appropriate, culturally sensitive breast cancer awareness and early detection program for women on the island. http://www.scielosp.org/scielo.php?script=sci_arttext&pid=S1020-49891999000300003
	Raju GC et al Breast cancer in West Indian women in Trinidad. Trop Geogr Med 1989;41(3):257-260
	Ronco A, De Stefani et al. Meat, fat and risk of breast cancer: a case-control study from Uruguay. Int J Cancer 65;328-331,1996
	Klabunde CN, Sancho-Garnier H, Taplin S, Thoresen S, Ohuchi N, Ballard-Barbash R; International Breast Cancer Screening Network.Quality assurance in follow-up and initial treatment for screening mammography programs in 22 countries. Int J Qual Health Care 2002;Dec14(6):449-61 OBJECTIVE: To describe the quality assurance activities related to follow-up evaluation of abnormal screening mammograms and subsequent initial treatment of women determined to have breast cancer for the screening programs represented in the International Breast Cancer Screening Network (IBSN). DESIGN: Analysis of data from a survey that included questions about screening program policies, standards, and procedures for follow-up of women with abnormal mammograms, as well as the data and measures that programs use to assess the adequacy of follow-up and initial treatment. SETTING AND PARTICIPANTS: IBSN representatives in 23 countries completed a comprehensive questionnaire between May and December 1998. RESULTS: Two-thirds of IBSN countries reported that they have a written policy or guidelines for follow-up of an abnormal mammogram; 64% require accreditation of the cytology or pathology laboratories that analyze breast specimens, or subject pathology laboratories to external audits. Of the 22 activities and measures related to quality of follow-up and initial treatment that we examined, all countries had in place at least half of them, although countries were more likely to have implemented activities and measures related to data collection and evaluation than to processes of care. CONCLUSIONS: Population-based screening mammography programs cannot achieve the goal of reducing breast cancer mortality if women with abnormal mammograms do not receive appropriate, timely follow-up and initial treatment. This study shows that IBSN countries vary in their implementation of procedures and measures to assure the quality of follow-up and initial treatment for women with abnormal screening mammograms. There is more emphasis on collecting and evaluating data than establishing mechanisms to ensure that the processes of care for follow-up and initial treatment are of high quality.
St. Kitts	Klabunde CN, Quality assurance in follow-up and initial treatment for screening mammography programs in 22 countries. Int J Quality in Health Care. 2002:15(1)449-461 Organized Breast screening service since 1996. 20% of target population

	screened. One registry. One facility. 2 Xray units. Linked to a cancer registry. There is no program to followup abnormal mammograms. There are no guidelines or policies for following up abnormal mammograms. They attempt to contact patients within 1 month of an abnormal mammogram. No minimum standards for ordering FNAC, Core Biopsy, Open biopsy. Once a mammogram is abnormal then the screening centre contacts the surgeon's office. Open biopsies are performed by surgeons or radiologists. Radiologists have to be certified for open biopsies. There are no accredited cytology labs. There is pathology lab accreditation. Pathology lab does not undergo external audit. The screening program has active access to cytology and pathology data. There is an assessment of recall rates. There are case conferences to review abnormal screens: involves radiologists, pathologist, surgeon. Assess the ratio of benign to malignant rates, Sens and Specificity. There is no specified breast cancer target rate on the first or subsequent screens. There is no assessment of interval cancer rates. There are no radiologic reviews of interval cancers. Available are surgeons, radiation docs, chemotherapy and hormone therapy. Tumor size sometimes assessed preop, always assessed at surgery, sometimes assessed by the pathologist. Nodes are always assessed by palpation and pathology.

SECTION 3 : EDUCATIONAL MATERIAL RELATED TO CERVICAL CANCER

To be included in this compendium the material was 1) developed by an international agency, or 2) if developed by a high resource setting there was evidence that it was assessed in a low resource setting or 3) available in languages other than English, and developed since the year 2000. The materials listed here are available in a variety of formats such as manuals, fast fact sheets, presentations, training manuals. Where materials are available in multiple languages we have indicated this.

Agency – indicates the host publisher.

Audience-the most likely group to benefit from being aware of this information

(c) – year the material was copyrighted

1. Educational Tools on Cancer Control Programs for Low Resource Settings

Agency	User	Item
WHO	Policy Makers	Cancer Control: Knowledge into action. WHO guide for effective programmes ©2006 http://www.who.int/bookorders/anglais/detart1.jsp?sesslan=1&codlan=1&codcol=15&codcch=674
NIH	Policy Makers	Disease Control Priorities in Developing Countries Chap 29: health Service Intervention for Cancer Control in developing Countries ©2006 http://www.ncbi.nlm.nih.gov/books/bv.fcgi?rid=dcp2.chapter.4129
WHO	Policy Makers	National Cancer Control Program: Policies and Managerial Guidelines. 2nd ed ©2002 http://www.who.int/cancer/media/en/408.pdf

2. Educational Tools on Breast Cancer from Prevention to Treatment

Agency	Audience	Web Line
CDC	Patient	Breast cancer http://www.cdc.gov/cancer/breast/basic_info/ *English and Spanish*
NCI	Physician	Breast Cancer - PDQ http://www.cancer.gov/cancertopics/types/breast
NCI	Public	Breast Cancer http://www.cancer.gov/cancertopics/types/breast *English and Spanish*
ACS	Public	Learn about Breast Cancer http://www.cancer.org/docroot/lrn/lrn_0.asp
CCS	Public	What is Breast Cancer http://www.cancer.ca/ccs/internet/standard/0,3182,3543_10175_273057_langId-en,00.html *English, French, Chinese, Farsi, Punjab*
Oncolink	Public	Breast Cancer http://www.oncolink.com/types/article.cfm?c=3&s=5&ss=33&id=8320
PATH	Health Care Providers, Policy Makers	Outlook: Breast Cancer: Increasing incidence, limited options http://www.path.org/files/eol19_4-rev.pdf *English, French, Chinese, Indonesian, Portuguese, Russian, Spanish*
AICR	Public	Breast Cancer http://www.aicr.org.uk/BreastCancerFAQs.stm
Susan Komer Foundation	Public	The ABC's of breast cancer prevention http://www.komen.org/intradoc-cgi/idc_cgi_isapi.dll?IdcService=SS_GET_PAGE&nodeId=472 *English and Spanish*

3. Educational Material on Screening

Agency	Audience	Web link
IARC		Breast Cancer Screening IARC Hanbook of Cancer Prevention, Volume 7 ISBN-13 9789283230076 ©2002 Breast cancer is the leading site of new cancer cases in women. Breast cancer detection is currently primarily based on physical examination by health care professionals, chance findings by women, breast self-examination and mammography used for diagnosis or for routine screening. Early enough detection through mass screening with mammography has been introduced in many countries in the hope that early intervention would lead to reduced mortality and less aggressive treatment. The aim of this publication is to provide an independent, authoritative review of the evidence of the efficacy and effectiveness of breast cancer screening. This will be of value to governments, public health officials and others concerned with policy recommendations for cancer control.

EMRO	Health Care Providers	Guidelines for the Early Detection and Screening of Breast Cancer ©2006 EMRO Technical Publications Series, No. 30 Khatib, O.M.N., Modjtabai, A. ISBN-13 9789290214069 Chapter 1 http://www.emro.who.int/ncd/publications/breastcancerscreening.pdf
ACS	patients	Cancer Facts for Women http://www.cancer.org/downloads/asn/CanFactsWom_Eng.pdf *English* http://www.cancer.org/downloads/ASN/CanFactsWom_Chin.pdf *Chinese* http://www.cancer.org/downloads/ASN/CanFactsWom_Kor.pdf *Korean* http://www.cancer.org/downloads/asn/CanFactsWom_Viet.pdf *Vietnamese*
NCI	Patients	NCI continued distribution and promotion of the half-hour television special and public service announcements on mammography "Una Vez al ano...Para toda una vida." The TV special was developed as a tool for educating Hispanic women on the need for breast cancer screening. "Una vez..." aired on the Univision Spanish- language television network for the second time during Breast Cancer Awareness Month in October 1993. Over 8,000 copies have been distributed to organizations serving the Hispanic population in the United States and Puerto Rico. The film is also being used widely by the Centers for Disease Control and Prevention Breast and Cervical Cancer Grantees, State Heath Departments, the Puerto Rico Department of Health, and by many units of the American Cancer Society.
WHO	Physicians	Fact Sheet http://www.who.int/cancer/detection/breastcancer/en/
ISNCC	Nurses	Yarbos CH. International Nursing and Breast Cancer The Breast journal. 2003;9:S2, S98-S100 Train the trainer 2 day course put on by ISNCC and Susan Komer Foundation. Participants included Brazil and Columbia as well as other countries. Not clear if an evaluation took place http://www.blackwell-synergy.com/doi/pdf/10.1046/j.1524-4741.9.s2.12.x
PAHO	Policy makers	Breast Cancer in Latin America and the Caribbean: Raising awareness or adopting costly programs? ©2002

4. Cytology

Agency	Audience	Resource
IARC	Pathology	Pathology and Genetics of Tumors of Breast and Female Genital Organs. ISBN 92 832 2412 4 ©2003 http://www.iarc.fr/WHO-BlueBooks/

5. *Biopsy Procedures*

Agency	Resource
American College of Surgeons	Stereotactic Breast Biopsy accreditation program http://www.facs.org/cancer/breastbiopprog.html

6. *Cancer Treatment*

Agency	Document
IARC	Guidelines for the Management of Breast Cancer EMRO Technical Publication Series, No. 31 ISBN-13 9789290214052 ©2006 Breast cancer remains a common and frequently fatal disease, the most commonly diagnosed cancer in women and the second leading cause of cancer death in the Eastern Mediterranean Region. Enhanced implementation of soundly developed, evidence-based treatment guidelines is an important goal for health services and individual clinicians. These guidelines have been developed to assist clinicians and patients to make decisions about treatment and thus improve health outcomes. They are intended to benefit oncologists, internists, secondary and tertiary hospitals, ministries of health and other health decision-makers in the Region. They provide the information necessary for decision-making by health care providers and patients themselves about the management of breast cancer.
EMRO	Guidelines for Management of Breast Cancer 1995 http://www.emro.who.int/dsaf/dsa510.pdf
ASCO	Recommendations for a core global curriculum in Medical Oncology http://www.jco.org/cgi/reprint/JCO.2004.08.134v1 *English, Chinese, Deutch, French, Italian, Japanese, Portuguese, Russian, Spanish*

7. *Palliative Care*

Focus	Audience	Resource and Link
Palliative Care	Health Care Providers	International Association for Hospital and Palliative Care manual of palliative care. http://www.hospicecare.com/manual/toc-main.html English
Cancer Pain	Health Care Provider	WHO Journal on issues related to cancer and pain control http://www.whocancerpain.wisc.edu/index.html
Palliation	Policy and Health Care Providers	Disease Control Priorities Project – Disease Control Priorities in Developing Countries: Chap 52-Pain Control for People with Cancer and AIDs http://www.ncbi.nlm.nih.gov/books/bv.fcgi?rid=dcp2.chapter.7766
Palliative care	Nurses	Curriculum for Palliative Nursing A core curriculum for a post basic course in palliative nursing © 2003 http://www.isncc.org/lists.asp?table=Publications#Core
ASCO	Health Care Providers	http://www.asco.org/portal/site/ASCO/menuitem.5d1b4bae73a9104ce277e89a320041a0/?vgnextoid=b1fbc2931f48d010VgnVCM100000ed730ad1RCRD

ACRONYMS

Short form	Definition
ACCP	Alliance for Cervical Cancer Prevention
ACS	American Cancer Society
AICR	American Institute for Cancer Research
AOGIN	Asia Oceania Research Organization on Genital Infection and Neoplasia
ASBD	Australasian Society for Breast Disease
ASCO	American Society of Clinical Oncology
ASHA	American Social health Association
ASTRO	American Society for Therapeutic and Readiation Oncology
CAP	College of American Pathologists
CCS	Canadian Cancer Society
CDC	Centre for Disease Control
EMRO	Eastern Mediterranean Research Organization
ESGO	European Society of Gynecologic Oncology
ESMO	European Society of Medical Oncology
ESTRO	European Society of Therapeutic Radiology and Oncology
EUROGIN	European Research Organization on Genital Infection and Neoplasia
EUSOMA	European Society of mastology
IAEA	International Atomic Energy Agency
IARC	International Agency for Research in Cancer
INCTR	International Network for Cancer Treatment and Research
ISBP	International Society of Breast Pathology
ISNCC	International Society for Nurses in Cancer Care
NCCC	National Cervical Cancer Coalition
NCI	National Cancer Institute
NIH	National Institute for Health
PACT	Programme of Action for Cancer Treatment
PAHO	PanAmerican Health Organization
PATH	Program in Advanced Technologies for Health
SGO	Society of Gynecologic Oncologists
UICC	International Union Against Cancer
USCAP	United States and Canadian Academy of Pathology
WHO	World Health Organization
WSBH	World Society for Breast Health

INDEX

D

J

L

M

N

S

T

U

V

W

Y